Chemical Ocular Burns

Norbert Schrage · François Burgher
Jöel Blomet · Lucien Bodson
Max Gerard · Alan Hall
Patrice Josset · Laurence Mathieu
Harold Merle

Chemical Ocular Burns

New Understanding and Treatments

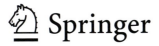

Authors

Norbert Schrage, MD

François Burgher, MD

Joël Blomet, MSc

Lucien Bodson, MD

Max Gérard, MD

Max Gérard, MD

Alan H. Hall, MD

Patrice Josset, MD

Laurence Mathieu, PhD

Harold Merle, MD

ISBN 978-3-642-14549-0   e-ISBN 978-3-642-14550-6

DOI 10.1007/978-3-642-14550-6

Springer Heidelberg Dordrecht London New York

Library of Congress Control Number: 2010937959

© Springer-Verlag Berlin Heidelberg 2011

This work is subject to copyright. All rights are reserved, whether the whole or part of the material is concerned, specifically the rights of translation, reprinting, reuse of illustrations, recitation, broadcasting, reproduction on microfilm or in any other way, and storage in data banks. Duplication of this publication or parts thereof is permitted only under the provisions of the German Copyright Law of September 9, 1965, in its current version, and permission for use must always be obtained from Springer. Violations are liable to prosecution under the German Copyright Law.

The use of general descriptive names, registered names, trademarks, etc. in this publication does not imply, even in the absence of a specific statement, that such names are exempt from the relevant protective laws and regulations and therefore free for general use.

Product liability: The publishers cannot guarantee the accuracy of any information about dosage and application contained in this book. In every individual case the user must check such information by consulting the relevant literature.

Cover design: eStudioCalamar, Figueres/Berlin

Printed on acid-free paper

Springer is part of Springer Science+Business Media (www.springer.com)

List of Authors

Norbert Schrage, MD Department of Ophthalmology of the City Hospital, Augenklinik Köln Merheim, 52070 Aachen, Germany
schrage@acto.de

François Burgher, MD PREVOR Laboratory, Moulin de Verville, 97760 Valmondois, France
fburgher@prevor.com

Joël Blomet, MSc PREVOR Laboratory, Moulin de Verville, 95760 Valmondois, France
jblomet@prevor.com

Lucien Bodson, MD CHU de Liège, Urgences-SAMU, Bat. 35, Sart Tilman par 4000, 1 Liège, Belgium
l.bodson@chu.ulg.ac.be

Max Gérard, MD Centre Hospitalier de Cayenne, Service d'Opthalmologie, 97306 Cayenne, Guyane, France
gerardmax@caramail.com

Alan H. Hall, MD TCMTS, Inc., The Benchmark Building, 1050 North 3rd street, Suite H, 82072 Laramie Wyoming, USA
ahall@toxic.com

Patrice Josset, MD Hôpital Trousseau, Laboratoire d'Anotomopathologie, Avenue du Dr. Arnold Netter 26, 75012 Paris, France
jossetpatrice@yahoo.fr

Laurence Mathieu, PhD Prevor Laboratory, Moulin de Verville, 95760 Valmondois, France
lmathieu@prevor.com

Harold Merle, MD CHU de Fort de France, Hôpital Pierre Zobda Quitman, 97261 Fort de France, Martinique
harold.merle@chu-fortdefrance.fr

Foreword

Despite rapid advances made in a number of medical fields for the last decades, chemical burns to the eye remain one of the most challenging ocular emergencies that eye doctors face today. Literature testifies that both the victim and the treating doctor have been plagued with frustration and disappointment even when a colossal of corrective measures have been taken during acute and chronic phases. This is because the outcome of chemical ocular burns is judged not solely by the completion of wound healing, a gold standard used in other medical subspecialties, but also by the recovery of normal vision. Inasmuch as successful wound healing is a desirable endpoint for emergency management of chemical ocular burns, the vision continues to be threatened and impeded by the resultant scarring.

Thus, it is exciting to witness the publication of a scientific book solely dedicated to such an important subject. In this book, Professor Norbert Scharge has assembled a group of experts specialized in chemistry, biochemistry, biology, epidemiology, emergency care, eye diseases, and surgical reconstruction to compile clinically useful and up-to-date knowledge related to chemical ocular burns. The contents are laid in a logical fashion and comprehensively and succinctly structured so that this book can be used as a handy reference for any acute care physician or eye doctor to gain an in-depth review before or during the management of such an eye emergency.

The book starts with a retrospective review of the history illustrating how chemical ocular burns had been managed in the past. The evolution of various treatment concepts and modalities discloses both human desperation and ingenuity. Intuitionally, the first goal of managing chemical ocular burns is to mitigate the extent of damage by instant elimination of the offending chemical (usually by irrigation with clean water or saline) so as to shorten its exposure. For the first time, this book makes a unique attempt to bridge the gap between basic chemistry and molecular pathogenesis by providing the scientific basis of how an exogenous chemical may alter biological materials at cellular and subcellular levels. Such information may allow researchers to uncover new therapeutic strategies not only to further negate but also to prophylactically avert the damaging effect. The latter notion is highly relevant in the wake of a future chemical warfare.

Upon halting the ongoing insult generated by exogenous chemicals, the conventional management has focused on ways to speed up wound healing so as to fend off potential infections. As eluded above, completion of wound healing often results in sight-threatening scar. To restore a useful vision, a number of surgical techniques including transplantation of limbal epithelial stem cells have been developed. These reconstructive surgeries have indeed brought back useful vision in a significant number of patients if an autologous source of limbal stem cells is employed. Nevertheless, the overall success is hampered if an allogeneic source is chosen for burns affecting both eyes unless a more vigorous systemic immunosuppression is instituted.

Therefore, pursuits should be continued to identify promising therapies to prevent cicatricial complications that inflict patients at the chronic phase. Emerging knowledge has told us that the wound healing is triggered by inflammation activated via innate immunity. Although the pathogenic basis remains elusive, all cicatricial complications due to chemical ocular burns are characterized by protracted and relentless inflammation. Several chapters of this book are devoted to providing enlightening glimpse into the mechanism thereby acute inflammation evolves into a chronic one. Such information has been useful for researchers to devise a new measure to abolish the progression of inflammation. One such potential therapy that has been put forth is transplantation of amniotic membrane as a biological bandage. When applied at the acute phase, i.e., within two weeks of burns, some moderately damaged eyes exhibit a remarkable recovery with rapid cessation of inflammation and few cicatricial complications. We begin realized that there is a golden window in which inflammation caused by chemical burns can be downregulated. Because such a novel intervention has resulted in notable tissue regeneration, chemical ocular burns may well be the ideal clinical arena where regenerative medicine can be practiced in the future.

Miami, Florida, USA   Scheffer C. G. Tseng

Preface

Whatever the origin of chemical burn lesions (i.e., whether resulting from a domestic accident, a chemical assault, or an industrial accident), such injuries can often result in serious functional visual injuries and significant physical and psychological consequences for the victims.

Nine authors of various disciplines and experiences have joined together to produce this book whose aim is to collectively present the most current and relevant data for each specific topic addressed.

As an introduction to the field of chemical ocular burn lesions, an historical and epidemiological perspective has been reviewed by an historian, an ophthalmologist, and a medical toxicologist. Next, a section is presented covering an expanded review of the mechanisms of action and reactivity of chemicals which can cause ocular injuries, prepared by a group of chemists and physicians.

A practicing ophthalmologist with additional experience in ocular physiology and histology then addresses fundamental and newly-developed methods for assessing ocular chemical burn injuries, particularly of the cornea, thus completing the discussion of the various mechanistic and pathophysiological aspects of ocular chemical burn lesions. Various methods for ocular chemical splash decontamination and the desirability of an efficacious active decontamination with the goal of preventing or minimizing ocular chemical burn injuries are discussed.

Following this are two sections prepared by practicing ophthalmologists which discuss clinical evaluation and current surgical treatment of ocular chemical burn injuries.

The book concludes with a section prepared by a chemist/physicist who conceived the innovative possibility of an active decontamination solution for ocular chemical splashes and an emergency physician who discuss specific decontamination measures and the emergent care of patients with ocular chemical burn injuries.

This work will prove useful for medical students, physicians-in-training, occupational medicine physicians and nurses, and private practice or hospital-based ophthalmologists, as well as for occupational health and safety personnel who deal with prevention and first aid measures for ocular chemical splashes, and who wish to supplement or update their understanding of ocular chemical burn injuries.

Gathering together all this technical knowledge introduces a new philosophy in the approach to chemical ocular burn lesions, in particular at the initial stage of victim management with increased practicality, specificity, and efficacy.

The multidisciplinary approach developed in this book also allows us, from the fundamental knowledge base, to envision other more diversified research on chemical burns in general.

The authors' goal is to promote the most beneficial care for patients with chemical ocular burn injuries by presenting the most precise and pertinent current information, and thus increasing communication and coordination between the various professionals involved in the prevention and treatment of such patients.

We are grateful to Oliver Mussate for translating this book from French to English.

Valmondois France   François Burgher

Contents

1 **History of Chemical Burns and Relative Treatments** 1
  Patrice Josset and Norbert Schrage

2 **Epidemiology of Ocular Chemical Burn Injuries** 9
  Alan H. Hall

3 **The Chemical Agents and the Involved Chemical Reactions** 17
  François Burgher, Laurence Mathieu, and Joël Blomet

4 **Histology and Physiology of the Cornea** 49
  Max Gérard and Patrice Josset

5 **Physiopathology of the Cornea and Physiopathology
  of Eye Burns** 59
  Norbert Schrage

6 **Rinsing Therapy of Eye Burns** 77
  Norbert Schrage

7 **The Clinical of Ocular Burns** 93
  Max Gérard

8 **Surgical Therapeutic of Ocular Burns** 103
  Harold Merle

9 **Emergency Treatment** 113
  Joël Blomet, Lucien Bodson, and Max Gérard

Index 119

History of Chemical Burns and Relative Treatments

Patrice Josset and Norbert Schrage

1.1 Burns for Doctors in Antiquity

The history of chemical burns and their relative treatments is still an unwritten chapter in the history of sciences. The present chapter aims to set up a framework of this history. We will first study the history of burns and their treatment from antiquity, before focusing on the treatment of chemical burns [1].

In Ancient Egypt, there were some recipes for the treatment of burns either in the critical phase or in the cicatricial phase and particularly a recipe to treat the ugly depigmentation of naturally tanned skins, daily exposed to a strong sun.

> Other remedy to prepare for a burnt zone, on first day: honey. Dress with it. Ebers 492 [2].
>
> "Other remedy for the conjuration of a burnt zone, on first day."
>
> (Dialog between a messenger and the goddess Isis)
>
> "Your son Heru is burnt in the desert. Is there any water there? There is no water. I have water in my mouth and the Nile between my thighs. I have come to extinguish the fire.
>
> Words to be spoken overt the breast milk of a woman who has borne a male child, gum, and ram's hair. This to be put on the burnt zone" Ebers 499
>
> "Other remedy (to eliminate white stains due to the burnt zone):
>
> Terebinth resin-Sntr 1 unit, honey 1 unit
>
> Anoint with this" Ebers 508

P. Josset (✉)
Anatomopathologist, "Armand Trousseau"
Children's Hospital, Paris, France
e-mail: patrice.josset@trs.ap-hop-paris.fr

N. Schrage
Department of Ophthalmology, Augenklinik
Köln Merheim, Cologne, Germany
e-mail: schrage@acto.de

Three thousand six hundred years ago, remedies such as honey and terebinth resin started to be used, and, since then, have been used all along history. The second recipe illustrates the mix of magic or religious practices and treatment.

As burns have always and very often occurred, most authors of Antiquity have written about them. Hippocrates has dealt with them in several writings and prescribed soothing substances and prevention from the cold. He has elaborated five formulae of medicines to prescribe for burns.

Much later, Guy de Chauliac (1298–1368) has written a few lines about burns in Chap. 6 of his surgery book (Fig. 1.1).

But the first author who has written about burns in a didactic way is Wilhelm Fabry von Hilden [3] (latine name: Fabricius Hildanus). In his essay, *de ambustionibus, quae oleo et aqua fervidis, ferro candente, pulvere tormentario, fulmine et quavis alia materia ignita fiunt*, written in Basel in 1607, the author classifies burns in three grades, and mentions the best treatment to apply for each case. He does not only prescribe a local treatment but also a general treatment, one of the goals of this latter being to prevent various complications. He gives indications on how to prevent the development of vicious scars. Wilhelm Fabry von Hilden seems to have been the first author to deal with burn treatment in a detailed and rational manner.

In the eighteenth century, Louis Laurent Heister (1683–1758) wrote a chapter about the study of burns in his "Institutions de chirurgie." He describes four grades of burns and prescribes the use of local treatments. He advises surgeons to look after the healing to prevent vicious scars.

In this century, various reflections about burns developed, particularly about the question of inner heat and nervous shock.

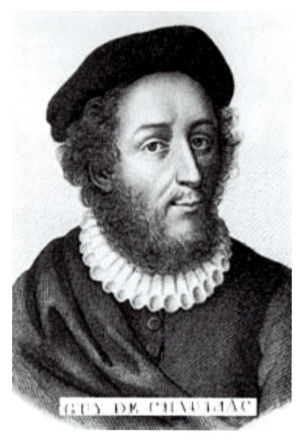

Fig. 1.1 Guy de Chauliac

In the nineteenth century, this point of view completely changed, and Guillaume Dupuytren [4] (1777–1835) through his lectures, either self-published or published by his numerous disciples, brought remarkable changes about this point. At first, he classified burns into five grades, the first three of which have the ability to spontaneously heal. He noticed the importance of the burnt surface and that patients with superficial but wide burns may die when others with deep but local burns survive. Early death is accompanied by weak pulsation, anuria, and breathing weakness. The point of the difficulty to evaluate the burnt surface was already studied in a book written by Alexis Boyer [5] (1757–1833), published in 1814. The author thinks that wide burns irritate the central nervous system and thus cause fever, infection, and death. For all authors, pain is a major element, although in case of deep burns, pain disappears, which was noticed by Lelong and Dupuytren in an essay published in 1819 [6].

Dupruyten thought that a quick death could not be due to an inflammatory reaction but was caused by a violent pain exhausting the nervous system, which made this death similar to a death due to a loss of big quantity of blood. He was remarkably brilliant in the treatment of the retractile sequelae of burns, which he knew how to treat with enough detachment from the critical phase. Indirectly [7], we also know that Dupruyten considered that the fragments of preserved healthy skin among burnt areas played a key role in healing.

Oliguria or anuria was highlighted by Auguste Nélaton (1807–1873) in his surgical pathology essay [8], in which he has also mentioned the deep thirst appearing soon after the first instances of the burn. The renal lesions were highlighted by Frederick Edward Obenaus in his 1847 essay [9] in which he also mentioned that blood looked viscous, sometimes coagulated in big vessels, and, in doing so, was similar to the blood obtained by practicing a bloodletting on burn victims. Consequently, it seemed that the losses of fluid provoked very important troubles of the organic functions, and that the loss of fluid through skin and mostly through burnt areas should be reduced as much as possible, and that blood should be diluted.

In 1855, the notion of crush kidney was developed by Ludwig von Buhhl (1816–1880) [10]. In parallel, the damages made to lungs were described by Gustav Passavant (1815–1893) on the occasion of the fire of a powder mill in Frankfurt am Main [11]. He then noticed that lungs could be hurt by heat, smoke, and toxic gas. That was a really premonitory vision of what would be recognized more than a century later.

In 1860, the histological lesions of the kidneys were described by Samuel Wilks in London but he did not consider them as the cause of patients' death [12].

Despite the exaggerated attention paid to general considerations such as pain in the causes of death, it became more and more evident that the general treatment was more important that the local one, at the end of the nineteenth century.

With a few variations, these considerations have supported the treatment of burn victims until the second half of the twentieth century. Then, it became finally possible to secure the general treatment of burns, which we will study below after a brief study of chemical burn since Antiquity (Fig. 1.2).

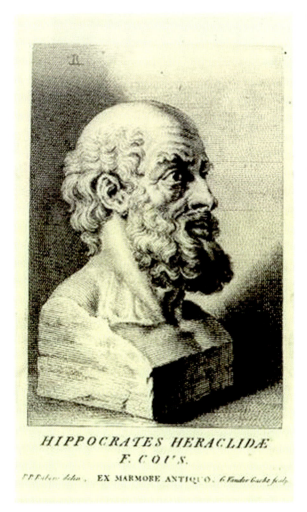

Fig. 1.2 Hippocrates Heraclidae

1.1.1 Chemical Burns Since Antiquity

It is not a surprise that there is no mention of chemical burn by antique authors such as Hippocrates, Galien, or Celse because the notion of chemical burn does not exist in their world; even cases of chemical burn might not have existed in their time.

Indeed, in Antiquity, substances or waters with acid or alkaline properties such as vinegar, lime, or alkaline products (soda, alkaline ashes) were well known but there was no mention of hurts specifically due to these substances. It is mentioned that some waters, particularly these from alkaline springs are not drinkable, but nothing more. Actually, it will take more than a thousand years so that concentrated acids and bases could be produced. Nevertheless, it is likely that accidents caused by lime have occurred.

The production of acids and bases is a direct consequence of the works of alchemists who did not start to work in the Middle Ages but in Hellenistic Alexandria [13]. So, from the twelfth to the sixteenth century, the following names appear: vitriol or sulfuric acid H_2SO_4, "eau forte" or nitric acid HNO_3, and "esprit de sel" or solution of hydrogen chloride (HCl) in water. The traditionally known bases such as potash, soda, or ammonia were called alkalis (from the Arabic word al-qâly designating the plants named soda).

In the twentieth century, the treatment of chemical burns becomes a bigger necessity during World War I. Combat gas burst into the battle provoking very severe lesions and a terrifying anxiety among fighters [14]. The town of Ypres (Ieper) in Belgium was one of the first towns contaminated by this combat gas on July 11, 1917, and thus has given the mustard gas its name as Yperite. This latter was then used in 1918 by the Germans in Verdun and "La Marne;" in 1919 by the British in Afghanistan; in 1925, on Winston Churchill's orders, by Britain on civil people in Kurdistan; in 1925 by France and Spain in Morocco; in 1934–1935 by Italy while it was occupying Ethiopia; in 1934–1944 by Japan against China; in 1963–1967 by Egypt in Yemen; and in 1983–1988, Saddam Hussein's regime used it against Kurd population in the north of Iraq. This mustard gas was also used during the war opposing Iraq and Iran.

As mentioned above, gas has been widely used and it is a powerful vesicant agent. In the form of vapor, it damages the respiratory tract. Eyes become temporarily blind and the skin in contact with the substance becomes inflammatory. The sweaty zones of skin are the most damaged as well as sensitive mucous membranes. If no treatment is applied, the cutaneous reaction provokes blisters full of liquid after 4–8 h. Spread in the form of particles, the gas penetrates the respiratory tract and destroys the mucous membranes with a respiration distress syndrome. Lungs suffer from emphysemae and edema due to the presence of fluids, which may cause a death similar to a drowning if the dose is too strong.

Finally, the patient suffers anemia, a drop of his immune resistance, and develops predispositions to cancers. Even when little concentrated, Yperite is indeed a mutagen agent.

It is easy to understand that, in this time, the treatment could only be purely symptomatic and only applied on skin and in absence of intense care, it could be qualified as "contemplative." When patients survived, their sequelae on skin were similar to those due to ordinary thermal or chemical burns. The ones suffering burns to the lungs often had a plus or minus serious definitive respiratory insufficiency.

Acid-base chemical accidents had already started earlier because of the industrial revolution but, as we know, the attention paid to the workers and risks on the workplace had been very deficient for a long time.

The only treatment, which is often revealed efficient enough, was the water washing of the chemical projections.

But, unfortunately, this was not always enough, particularly for eyes burns, because of the ocular epithelium being extremely fragile, or in case of wide burns or burns due to specific substances such as hydrofluoric acid.

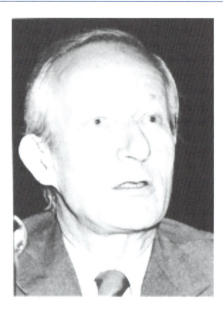

Fig. 1.3 Marcel Legrain

1.1.2 Treatment of Thermal and Chemical Burns in the Second Half of Twentieth Century, the Revolution of Intensive Care

The very difficult situation of burnt patients lasted at least till the 1960s. It was deeply modified after the works and realizations of Prof. Marcel Legrain (1923–2003) (Fig. 1.3) who was the pioneer of renal physiology, and particularly of acute renal failure that he studied in the 1940s and 1950s. He went to Boston for two years and afterward he opened the first unit of renal dialysis, in Hotel Dieu Hospital in Paris. His disciples Aubert and Saisy opened the first center of Dialysis in Choisy Clinic and Saizy opened a Centre of Anaesthesia treating burnt patients in St Antoine Hospital in Paris. From Prehistory, the situation had evolved to accurate intensive cares that could compensate the huge losses of severe burned patients.

Scientists and doctors could thus discover hydroelectrolytic, caloric (up to 1,000 calories/day), endocrinous, and other losses.

Then the techniques by Saisy and his colleagues have widely spread in France, enabling a more and more efficient symptomatic treatment of burnt patients. Here, we won't study the points about surgery of burnt patients and skin transplantations.

Complicated by military secret, the issue of chemical war is still present today. For sure, the great powers have made big efforts to develop bacteriological and chemical weapons, among which are the neurotoxic agents. American soldiers suffering Gulf war syndrome may suffer consequences of this chemical pollution (because of the uranium and toxic substances released by bombing on Iraqi sites close to American soldiers). The secret about the production and nature of burns caused by chemical weapons confront doctors with strange burns and the collaboration between doctors (particularly between several countries) is in opposition with military actions. We shall remind that on February 6, 1918, [14] the Red Cross asked the belligerents not to use asphyxiating or deleterious gases, which with many other acts is to be credited to this institution and its founder, Henri Dunant.

A major progress toward the recognition of chemical burns was the recognition of pulmonary chemical burns, a discovery in which the Burns Surgery Department of St Antoine Hospital played an important part. Actually, the role of pulmonary burns due to chemicals had been unrecognized for a long time. Nevertheless, observers noticed that after 2 or 3 days victims of fire smokes might develop serious lung pathology, which was often lethal. The use of bronchial fibroscopies helped to authenticate the lesions of the mucous membrane and the highlighting of numerous chemically active toxic substances in the fire smokes enables the assertion of the reality of the entity and helps to understand its mechanism.

1.1.3 History of the Treatment of Chemical Skin Burns

For a long time, the only applied and applicable treatment of chemical burns was water washing. The importance of the time passed between burn and the washing was an evidence. In front of the importance of pain and lesions, the idea of neutralization came out using the following reaction

$$Acid + Base \rightarrow Salt + Water$$

but it was soon noticed that the treatment was not perfect because it required a balance of one to one molecule of the reagents and the exothermic character of the reaction was ignored.

So, the treatment of an acid burn by a base resulted in the following reaction

Acid + excess of base → salt + base + heat with following results

- Possibly an acid burn due to the first instants of contact
- An alkali burn
- A thermal burn!

What an ambivalent result!

Before the little convincing result of this treatment, it became recommended to wash only with current water.

From the 1970s, the introduction of tampon solutions or amphoteric solutions, particularly in France and Germany, was quite difficult because of the legislation, which would not include specific cases. Particularly in France, it was difficult to convince the doctors of the interest of amphoteric solutions, which did not let heat out, but brought the skin or eye to a neutral pH and left no acid or alkali residue. This situation was partly due to a weak knowledge of chemistry in the medical world, whereas it was easier to convince chemists. Anyway, the use of amphoteric solutions has little by little spread into the industrial world and lead to some exciting results. In opposition to previous reasoning, it was noticed that the use of such solutions could have a positive effect even in case of late application. It is then necessary to develop a more and more universal solution that could neutralize a lot of chemical agents, as well as it is necessary to develop more specific solutions.

1.1.4 Conclusion

The history of the treatment of burns was first made of a long period from Antiquity to the first half of the twentieth century, during which men tried to do their best and understand the mechanisms of local burn and general symptoms from the nineteenth century. Intensive care has revolutionized the treatment and survival of burnt patients. There is a lot to expect from the future not only because of the possible development of solutions that can neutralize chemical agents and because of the improvement of the intensive care techniques, but also because of the improvement of the skin transplantation techniques or eye surgical methods and of the treatment of lesions due to gas breathing, the mortality of which is still very high and for which it will be necessary to imagine neutralization and decontamination using a spray as soon as possible.

1.2 Modern History of the Chemical Burns

Eye burns are an old phenomenon and have been described as soon as high temperature and small amounts of concentrated liquids were available. In Antiquity, it was a common procedure to damage eyes for punishment or for assault as described in the Old Testimony.

In the Middle Ages, there were only a few historical descriptions of eye burns from hot fluids and chemicals.

1.2.1 Burns, a Disease of Different Origins

The differentiation between chemical burns and thermal burns has first been made by ophthalmologists in the early 1920s of the last century. Poor prognosis and early primary enucleation were due to the lack of therapeutic alternatives and resulted in devastating outcomes at this time.

1.2.2 Start of Medical Treatment

First systematic work rose in the highly industrialized areas of Europe when ophthalmologists were facing a lot of patients exposed to splashes of highly corrosive substances. One of the first books specialized in this topic that addressed the special problems of those patients was "Augenschäedigungen in Industrie und Gewerbe," written by Jaensch in 1958. Jaensch was a German ophthalmologist recognizing the interaction of occupational medicine, ophthalmology, and toxicology. He lived in the area of Düsseldorf, where there were a lot of chemical and metal industry plants. Starting with lid corrections, conjunctival surgery and intraocular glaucoma and cataract surgery, the emerging possibilities of anterior segment surgery has provided the first opportunities of improvement of the prognosis of these devastating diseases. Except this experiment, within the following decades, eye burns did not interest the researchers as eye burns but only served as a model of non-healing inflammatory disease.

1.2.3 Research in Toxicology and Ophthalmology

First systematic therapeutic strategies were introduced by Passow [15, 16] who recommended rinsing with water and releasing the toxic secret from the conjunctiva via the "Passow incisions." Later on Thiel [17, 18] in Frankfurt published his work on decontamination of the burnt eye with buffers and first approached the healing of the chronic inflammation. After World War II, some young researchers tried to identify the chronic inflammation after eye burns as a crucial problem and as a fruitful field of research to address a lot of specific diseases of the eye. The test model being introduced in this field was the Draize test, which since the late 50s of the last century has served as a toxicological evaluation of chemicals, drugs, and cosmetics to be approved by the regulatory bodies in America and Europe.

1.2.4 Rinsing Therapy

Beside the medical interest, the first pharmaceutical companies have offered specific solutions and installations to rinse the burnt eye. To the early recommendations of rinsing with water were added the recommendations to use phosphate buffer from Laux [19–21] whose ideas have been set up by the Winzer Company in Germany. Other recommendations were to use borate or diluted acetate solutions sold in France by a pharmaceutical enterprise directed by Jacques Blomet. In the USA, the systematic treatment and prevention program in health and occupational work started in 1959 with firms such as FendAll distributing phosphate buffer solutions. The rinsing solutions gave first efficient treatment options and a lot of severe eye burns could be prevented by the use of water and buffers.

Training and education of workers in exposed areas became a standard procedure, but the number of chemicals, their concentrations, and their use spread faster than safety developments improved, so that within the 1970s the number of victims of eye burns reached a peak in the industrialized world.

1.2.5 Classification of Eye Burns

A new systematic approach started with the classification of eye burns introduced by Roper Hall in 1978, giving hints from the initial clinical presentation to the later outcome. The modified classification from Reim reflected the observation that limbus affection and circulation in the limbus area in the early posttraumatic phase gives major information on the later outcome of eye burns.

Thus, Reim et al. introduced early treatment options for eye burns starting with a concept of corneal opacity, limbal ischemia, and conjunctival damage. Thus a prognostic and therapeutic concept existed that made the prognosis more certain. Modifications of this concept are all based on this fundamental work.

1.2.6 Specific Treatment Options

First the recognition of severe ischemia as a result of the eye burn was addressed by emerging vasodilatators like Priscol that was proposed and used by Nagy F. [22] (Ophthalmologica Basel 121, 1951, 345). A systematic eye burn research started with some people related to the Boston Cornea Foundation around persons like Roswell Pfister, Chris Dohlmann, Martin Reim, and Christopher Paterson. They all first focused on different parts of clinical evaluation of eye burns. Roswell Pfister looked for intermediate phase treatment concepts with mediator, metabolic, and histological definitions of the problem. Martin Reim focused on metabolic disorders, new surgical options, and corneal transplantation after eye burns, whereas his friend J. Friend focused on elementary biochemical issues. Mostly coming from biochemistry, Chris Dohlmann found the devastating eye burns worth to develop a keratoprosthesis, which has been implanted from then on up to today. Last but not the least out of this working group was Christopher Paterson who focused on first aid, intraocular pressure, and treatment with vitamin C and citrate together with RR Pfister. Nevertheless, all of those researchers found the chronic inflammation and the treatment options in theoretical and practical approach to be an interesting scientific and clinical topic.

Systematic research in treating started with modification of the synthesis of collagens by high doses of vitamin C introduced by Reim, Pfister, and Paterson and citrate treatment introduced by Pfister. Surgical improvements with Passow's incisions, and Thiel's peridectomy and improved plastic lid surgery increased the healing chances. The enthusiasm to control ongoing inflammation in eye burns being introduced by topical and systemic corticosteroids in the 1970s lead to improvements but clinicians were disappointed that severe scars, disabling corneal opacities and severe glaucoma were out of control in severe cases. Improvements of other disciplines in ophthalmology like glaucoma valves, keratoprosthesis, transplantations under immunosuppression, and stem cell transplants were used in parallel to the rise of those new techniques. Today an equilibrated concept of modern first aid with amphoteres, steroids, vitamin c, antibiotic, and defined surgical techniques is the common repertoire of specialists in the field of ocular reconstruction after eye burns. Thus in the last 10 years, we have not lost one eye from eye burns, which in comparison to the old times is a great success. Surgical techniques now aim to restore sight which we do not achieve in all cases today. Major improvements like the longtime forgotten amnion technique from de Rüther and others in 1990 result in enormous improvement of the therapeutic reservoir of modern ophthalmology.

1.2.7 Future and Present of Reconstitutive Concepts

Mostly Prof. Sh Tseng with his stem cell concept in transplantation should be mentioned as a protagonist of the "new world" of concepts with adult stem cells opening the door for future concepts reaching in the horizon of today performed stem cell proliferation and seeding provided by Pellegrini et al. The future of stem cell concepts with reformation of individual stem cells by gene therapy or other techniques might solve the severe problems in eye burns in future. Nevertheless, the first gleam of hope for artificial corneas rose with research of reconstituted endothelium from K. Engelmann and M. Böhnke as well as from the group around May Griffith who tried to reconstitute human three-dimensional models.

References

1. History of the treatment of burns. Burns (Suppl 1), S1–S46 (1988)
2. Thierry, B.: les papyrus médicaux de l'Égypte pharaonique. Fayard, Paris (1995)
3. Heister, Institutions de chirurgie, traduit du latin par M Paul, Paris, 1771, livre II, chap. XVI
4. Dupuytren, G.: Leçons cliniques sur les brûlures. Clinique Par 2, 83–85, 89–90, 138–140 (1830); Coubret, J.-B.: Dissertation sur les brûlures. Paris (1813); Marsal, J.B.A.: Dissertation sur les effects et le traitement de la brulure. Paris (1812); Moulinié, J.: Brûlures. Paris (1812)
5. Boyer, J., Guinard, L.: Des brûlures causes des troubles fonctionnels et accidents généraux qu'elles déterminent. Etude et recherches expérimentales, Paris (1895)
6. Lelong, F.: Dissertation sur les brûlures. Paris (1819)
7. Mainot, P.V.: Essai sur la brûlure. Paris (1830)
8. Nélaton, A.: Eléments de pathologie chirurgicale, vol I, pp. 285–303. Paris (1844)
9. Obenaus, C.F.E.: De combustione cutanea eiusque effectu lethifero. Leipzig (1847)

10. Buhl, Mittheilungen aus des Pfeuferschen Klinik, Epidemische Cholera, Ztschr. f. rat. Med. n.F. 6,77
11. Passavant, G.: Bemerkungen über Verbrennungen des menschlichen Körpers und deren Behandlung mit dem permanenten warmen Bade. Deutsche Klinik Berl 10, 365–366, 373–375 (1858)
12. Wilks, S.: On some diseases of children. Guy's Hosp Rep Lond 3 S 6, 101–148 (1860)
13. Berthelot, M.: les Alchimistes grecs. Paris (1888)
14. http://www.icrc.org/Web/fre/sitefre0.nsf/html/5FZGZT
15. Passow, A.: Early operation performable in ambulant practice in therapy and prevention of corneal lesions and necrosis in burns of the eye. Klin Monatsblatter Augenheilkd Augenarztl Fortbild 127(2), 129–142 (1955). German (No abstract available)
16. Passow, A.: Early operation in chemical and thermal injuries to get rid of the toxic products; experience with eye and skin. Med Klin (Munich) 51(8), 293–297 (1956). German
17. Thiel, H.L.: Treatment of caustic eye burns. Med Monatsschr 12(8), 542–544 (1958). German
18. Thiel, H.L.: Proceedings: The treatment of eye injuries (author's transl). Langenbecks Arch Chir 334, 429–434 (1973)
19. Laux, U.: The water pic instrument for immediate intensive irrigation of the eye at the place of accident. Zentralbl Arbeitsmed Arbeitsschutz Prophyl 26(10), 215–220 (1976). German
20. Laux, U., Roth, H.W.: Intensive irrigation of the eye in lime burns by means of pulsating water stream (author's transl). Klin Monatsbl Augenheilkd 165(4), 664–669 (1974). German
21. Laux, U., Roth, H.W., Krey, H., Steinhardt, B.: Aqueous humor pH in experimental lye burns and influence of different treatment measures (author's transl). Albrecht Von Graefes Arch Klin Exp Ophthalmol 195(1), 33–40 (1975). German
22. Nagy, F.: Priscol therapy of corrosions and burns of the eye. Ophthalmologica 121(6), 345–352 (1951)

Epidemiology of Ocular Chemical Burn Injuries

Alan H. Hall

2.1 Introduction

Ocular chemical burns are a significant problem [1] because they may destroy the entire corneal epithelium and extend into the fornices [2]. More than 25,000 chemical products – oxidizers, reducing agents, corrosives, etc. – have the potential to cause chemical burns [3]. Because serious eye burns can result in loss of sight or require corneal transplants, such chemical burns must be taken seriously.

2.2 Data Limitations and Scope of the Problem

No international or national databases were found that specifically collect data on ocular chemical injuries. There are individual publications detailing burns in general or chemical burns (including eye and/or skin burns) in a region or country and case series from burn centers, hospitals, or groups of hospitals. Occupational burn data are usually regional in nature or are case series. National Poison Center databases such as the US American Association of Poison Centers' National Poison Data System (NPDS) collect data on the annual number of eye exposures, but do not contain specific information regarding the specific chemical substance(s) involved, the type of initial decontamination, the time from exposure to initial decontamination, and clinical outcomes. National occupational exposure databases such as the US Department of Labor Statistics (BLS) also contain only nonspecific data and also do not collect specific information regarding the specific chemical substance(s) involved, the type of initial decontamination, the time from exposure to initial decontamination, and clinical outcomes. Information such as the number of lost work days, number of eye injuries, industry segment, and rates of injury per 10,000 full-time workers from the US BLS data do provide some insights into the scope of the problem.

2.2.1 Individual Publications/Case Series

Josset et al. [4] found that there were approximately 7,000 serious chemical splash injuries in France per year, with about half of these cases involving the eyes [4]. Chemical eye splashes made up about 9.9% of ocular trauma in the USA and 7.2% in a UK casualty department; however, most were with rather innocuous substances such as hairsprays and shampoos [5]. Acid and base eye burns were 1.6% and 0.6%, respectively, of total eye injuries [5].

Ocular burns comprise about 7–18% of ocular trauma presenting to emergency departments in the USA and eye injuries account for about 3–4% of total occupational injuries [6]. Most of these (approximately 84%) are chemical burns. About 15–20% of patients with facial burns also have ocular burns. The ratio of acid/alkali chemical ocular burns is 1:1–1:4 [6].

A.H. Hall
TCMTS, Inc., Laramie, WYOMING, USA, and
Colorado School of Public Health, Denver,
Colorado, USA
e-mail: ahalltoxic@msn.com

In a 5-year retrospective study of 383 patients with eye injuries (397 eyes involved) in Croatia, 13.6% sustained chemical injuries [7]. Of the total patients with burned eyes, 54 required hospital admission [7]. A 7-year retrospective study of 60 hospitalized cases of pediatric eye injuries in Hong Kong found that 10% were ocular chemical burns [8].

In a US study of compensable work-related ocular injuries, the incidence of eye burns was 23.4 per 10,000 employees [9]. The majority of these were associated with chemical exposures.

In a retrospective study of 148 cases of occupational eye injuries in Germany, ocular burns (not specified as chemical or other etiology) comprised 15.5% of the total [10]. In another German study of 101 patients with 131 severely burned eyes, 72.3% of the injuries were work-related, 84.2% were chemical injuries, and 79.8% of these were due to alkalis [11]. Of the 42 cases of alkali ocular burns admitted to a German eye clinic between 1985 and 1992, 73.8% involved industrial accidents [11]. In Finland in 1973, 11.9% of all industrial accidents were ocular injuries and burns comprised 3.6% of these (chemical or other injury mechanism not specified) [12].

A 7-year retrospective Australian study of 182 industrial burns found that 5.5% were ocular burns due to chemicals, gas explosions, and electric flashes (percentages not specified) [13]. In another Australian study of 159 cases of hospital-admitted alkali ocular burn patients from 1972–1981, the majority of burns were Grade 1 or 2 and none of these resulted in vision loss [14].

In contrast, in a US Poison Center study of a random sampling of 500 cases of chemical eye exposure over a 6-month period in 1986, the majority (84.4%) occurred in the home and involved household products [15]. These most commonly involved accidental exposures in children [15].

2.2.2 American Association of Poison Centers National Poison Data System (NDPS)

Data on poison exposures reported to US Poison Centers are collected on a daily basis and published yearly in the American Association of Poison Centers National Poison Data System (NPDS) Annual Report [16]. In the latest published report for the year 2006, there were 2,403,539 human poison exposure cases, including 136,534 eye exposures (5.4%), with 2 deaths [16].

2.2.3 US Bureau of Labor Statistics Data

The US Bureau of Labor Statistics collects data annually regarding workplace injuries. The latest data at the time of this writing are from 2006. While these data are quite nonspecific and difficult to relate directly to the epidemiology of ocular chemical injuries, they do provide some insight into the scope of the problem. All of the following data refer to *private industry* and *cases of nonfatal injuries or illnesses resulting in lost work days*.

The incidence rate in 2006 for chemical burns (not specified as to eye and/or skin) was 1 per 10,000 full-time workers and the median number of lost work days was 3 [17]. There were 7,490 chemical burns (also not specified as to eye and/or skin). Eye injuries and illness totaled 35,970 with the largest number, 17,760 (49%), occurring in the Total Goods industry segment [17]. The industry segment, Chemicals and Chemical Products, accounted for 19,480 occupational injuries or illnesses, with the largest number, 19,480 (65%), occurring in the Total Service Providing industry segment.

Overall, chemical burns comprised 0.6% of total occupational injuries and illnesses resulting in lost work time and chemicals and chemical products accounted for 1.6 % of such injuries or illnesses [17]. The incidence of chemical burns (not specified as to eye and/or skin) was 0.8 per 10,000 full-time workers. The incidence rate for the Chemicals and Chemical Products industry segment was 2.1 per 10,000 full-time workers.

The percent distribution of lost work days in the Chemicals or Chemical Products industry segment was as follows [17]:

Lost work days	Percent
1 day	28.8%
2 days	19.0%
3–5 days	24.7%
4–20 days	7.6%
21–30 days	2.4%
31 days or more	7.8%

2.3 Etiology

2.3.1 Work-Related Injury

Of 1,720 persons with occupational burn injuries in the US State of North Carolina, the most common event was exposure to corrosive substances [18]. Of burn injury patients from all causes, 361 patients (69.6%) also had eye burns [18]. Ocular burns comprise about 7–18% of ocular trauma presenting to emergency departments in the USA and eye injuries account for about 3–4% of total occupational injuries [6]. Most of these (approximately 84%) are chemical burns. About 15–20% of patients with facial burns also have ocular burns. The ratio of acid/alkali chemical ocular burns is 1:1–1:4 [6].

In a retrospective study of 148 cases of occupational eye injuries in Germany, ocular burns (not specified as chemical or other etiology) comprised 15.5% of the total [10]. In another German study of 101 patients with 131 severely burned eyes, 72.3% of the injuries were work-related, 84.2% were chemical injuries, and 79.8% of these were due to alkalis [11]. Of 42 cases of alkali ocular burns admitted to a German eye clinic between 1985 and 1992, 73.8% involved industrial accidents [19]. In Finland in 1973, 11.9% of all industrial accidents were ocular injuries and burns comprised 3.6% of these (chemical or other injury mechanism not specified) [12]. A 7-year retrospective Australian study of 182 industrial burns found that 5.5% were ocular burns due to chemicals, gas explosions, and electric flashes (percentages not specified) [30]. In a 4-year hospital-based study in Taiwan, of 486 patients with eye injuries, 39.9% were work-related [20]. Chemical ocular burns accounted for 19.6% of these injuries [20].

2.3.2 Deliberate Chemical Assault

"The challenge in such cases is to save the eyes…" [21]. Beare [22] reported a series of 64 patients with eye injuries from chemical assaults treated in a specialty eye hospital in London with 20,333 Accident and Emergency Department visits and 29,853 outpatient visits during a 12-month period in 1988 [22]. In 17 eyes of 16 patients, there was a total loss of corneal epithelium with varying degrees of limbal ischemia. Nine eyes were essentially blinded and two eyes had less severe but permanent vision loss.

There had been a marked increase in the number of patients presenting to this hospital with chemical eye injuries from assaults over a 6-year period beginning in 1984, when only 1 case was seen [22]. There were 3 cases in 1985, 15 cases in 1986, 37 cases in 1987, and 40 cases in 1988. Of the 64 reported patients, 55 were male and 9 were female. Six patients also had significant facial or eyelid burns, although none became necrotic. Assailants were often gangs of male youths in their teens to twenties, and racial bias was a likely precipitant in certain cases.

Thirty-seven patients (58%) had a unilateral eye injury and 27 (42%) had bilateral injuries, for a total of 91 injured eyes [22]. The chemical agent involved was generally unknown, although 6 patients reported smelling ammonia. The time between exposure and initial water irrigation ranged from 5 s to 2 h, with irrigation usually on three separate occasions: first by the victim with tap water, second with normal saline in the Accident and Emergency Department, and third with potassium dehydrogenate orthophosphate buffered solution in distilled water at the specialty eye hospital.

The conjunctival sac pH was measured with test paper and was alkaline in 46 eyes (51%) (pH 7.0–9.0), neutral in 4 eyes (4%), acidic in one eye (1%) and was not recorded in the remaining 40 eyes [22]. In 16/91 (19%) of injured eyes, there were varying degrees of limbal ischemia. The majority of injured eyes (73%) were Grade I (minimal) on the Roper-Hall grading system. Six eyes (7%) were grade II injuries, two (2%) were Grade III injuries, and nine (10%) were Grade IV injuries. Marked conjunctival stromal edema was seen in all Grade III and IV injured eyes, and evidence of chemical damage to the anterior lens capsule was present in the nine most severely injured eyes. Hypopyon occurred in four eyes.

Thirty-one patients were admitted to hospital for an average of 3.3 days (range: 1–14 days) [22]. The approximate cost of treatment was £500.00 per patient.

The eight most severely injured patients (15%) with Grade IV injuries had gross scarring, vascularization, and a permanent severe reduction in vision, bilateral in one case [22]. There were two cases of infectious keratitis with *Staphylococcus aureus* in patients with persistent corneal epithelial defects; this progressed to globe perforation in one case. One patient underwent corneal grafting 20 months post-injury. None of the 64 patients developed symblepharon, but 1 patient with severe injuries was registered as blind [22].

O'Driscoll et al. [23] briefly reported several patients with severe ocular injuries presenting to a specialty eye hospital in Birmingham, UK over a several week period [23]. These patients had been deliberately splashed with alkaline substances (not specified) during robberies or violent assaults. The assailants were most often children or young adults. These authors note that alkali eye injuries involve massive corneal and conjunctival epithelial loss and that necrosis of the corneal stem cells can develop, resulting in delayed healing with scarring. Secondary glaucoma may develop. The alkali injured eye may be irreversibly damaged and a painful, blind eye may result [23].

In his discussion, Beare [22] compared the above UK series to a series reported from the USA by Klein and Lobes (1984) [22]. In the US series, of 52 patients reported, assault was the cause in 35 cases with the assailants being women and the victims being men. Severe burns were frequently present, with 39% of 100 injured eyes being classified as very severely damaged on the Hughes scale. In this US series, 58% of injured eyes had a final visual acuity of less than 20/20. There was a globe perforation rate of 13/100 (13%) in these injured eyes. The incidence of symblepharon was 29% and that of secondary glaucoma was 18% in this US series [22].

Yeong et al. [24] reported 15 cases of facial mutilation from chemical assaults from 1991 to 1992 in Taiwan [24]. There were 10 women and 5 men and 10/15 (66%) identified the assailant. In 6/15 cases, the assailant was the spouse.

Ninety percent of victims claimed that sulfuric acid was the chemical involved [24]. Injured areas were confined to the head and neck. While most had their faces flushed with tap water, none had continuous effective flushing, especially of the eyes, before presentation to hospital. Most had half or more of their faces grossly disfigured by scars. Six patients (40%) had total bilateral blindness and one had partial loss of vision. Other common function sequelae were: lower eyelid ectropion (14/15), microstomia (12/15), cervical flexion contracture (10/15), ear deformity (8/15), and nostril stenosis (6/15). Victims had severe psychological and social effects, and most lived as recluses.

In their discussion, Yeong et al. [24] described four case series of chemical assaults from the USA, two from New York City, one from Washington DC, and one from Dallas, Texas [24]. In New York City, Crikelair et al. [25] reported that 15 of the 145 patients admitted to the burn center of one hospital had sustained chemical assaults [24]. All 15 cases involved a mixture of household lye mixed with water. Permanent visual loss occurred in three victims.

Amongst a series of 38 victims of chemical assault (acids) in Bangladesh, 10 (26%) had injuries of the eyeballs and 18 (47%) had injury of the eyelids [26]. Merle et al. [27] studied 66 patients with alkali ocular burns (104 eyes) in Martinique (French West Indies) over a 4-year period, of which nearly half (45.5%) were due to deliberate chemical assault (the most frequently involved product was Alkali®; 15.3% ammonia, pH 12.8) [27].

Branday et al. [28] reported that 562 patients with acute chemical injuries were admitted to 8 regional hospitals in Jamaica during a 10-year period from 1981–1990 [28]. Chemical burns comprised 13.3% of all burn patients admitted during this time period. Nearly half (236 cases 42%) of these chemical burns resulted from deliberate assault, while only 10 of the total chemical burn cases (1.8%) were the result of work-related accidents. In one of the study hospitals, 38% of burn admissions were due to chemical burns and 2/3 of these were due to deliberate chemical assaults. Assailants were more likely to be female and victims were either male or other women over disputes involving a relationship with a male partner [28].

Of the overall chemical burn patients, the most common sites involved were the face, neck, and upper body (87%), and the eyes or eyelids were involved in 19% of overall cases [28]. In deliberate chemical assault victims, the face and neck were commonly injured, but the genital area was also involved in many victims. Acids, such as sulfuric acid, can be obtained at low cost in Jamaica. These authors note that many of the chemical assault injuries were devastating with facial destruction and blindness. Less than half of the victims decontaminated themselves with copious water irrigation before presenting to hospital [28].

Asaria et al. [29] reported a retrospective review of 125 burn patients admitted to a hospital in Kampala, Uganda over an 18-month period in 2001–2002 [29]. Of these, 15 patients (17%) were victims of deliberate acid assault. The male/female ratio was 1:1. The average total body surface area (TBSA) involved was 14.1% and the most common burn sites were the face (86.7%), head and neck (66.7%), chest (53.5%), and upper limbs (60%). The eyes were commonly involved

(33.3%) and victims experienced partial or complete blindness. Fourteen of the 15 patients (93.3%) had permanent scarring as sequelae and 7 (46.7%) of them developed cervical or axillary contractures. Other significant sequelae included ectropion (33.3%), nostril stenosis (13.3%), microstomia (20.0%), paraphimosis (6.7%), and Cushing's ulcers (6.7%) [29].

The circumstances of the acid assault involved attacks by unknown assailants during a robbery in 46.7% (26.7% during a car or motorcycle robbery and 20.0% in a house robbery). A known person was the assailant in 33% of these acid assaults, commonly in a setting of marital discord. Many of these patients ended up living as recluses and dependent on family members for daily support. The acid involved in most cases was sulfuric acid used to restore exhausted automobile batteries, which is readily available at low cost from garages in Uganda [29].

Saini and Sharma [30] reported 145 eye injuries amongst 102 Indian patients treated at a major referral center [30]. There were only seven chemical assault victims, but the authors noted that these patients had more severe injuries than patients with accidental injuries with 71.4% of the eyes of chemical assault victims developing phthis bulbi (a deformed eyeball with no light perception). In contrast, phthis bulbi developed in only 3.6% of patients with accidental chemical exposures [30].

Non-governmental organizations (NGOs) play an important role in the management of victims of deliberate chemical assaults. For example, in Bangladesh the Acid Survivors Foundation (ASF) provides assistance with medical and surgical treatment [37], legal aid, and rehabilitation through a social program of training and employment assistance. The NGO also works on programs for prevention and for decreasing the delay to decontamination and access to medical treatment by establishing new facilities in rural areas.

2.3.3 Complications of Face Peeling

Severe burning sensation, redness, epiphora of the left eye, mild upper eyelid edema of the right eye, severe edema of the left eyelids, left eye inferior ectropion, blepharoconjunctivitis with severe hyperemia, papillary reaction, and chemosis occurred in a patient undergoing a face peeling procedure with a trichloroacetic acid-containing mask [31].

A 47-year-old woman undergoing face peeling with 35% trichloroacetic acid developed left eye burning sensation, excessive tearing, marked conjunctival injection, conjunctival infection, and mild inferior superficial punctuate keratitis involving 25% of the cornea [32].

2.3.4 Burn Center/Hospital Studies

Amongst 377 patients with chemical burns admitted to a burn center in Guangdong province, China from 1987–2001, 337 (88.5%) were accidental and 40 (10.5%) were from deliberate chemical assault [33]. Of the total number of chemically burned patients, ocular burns occurred in 55 (14.6%) [33].

Saini and Sharma [30] reported a series of 145 chemical eye injuries in 102 patients treated at a major referral center in India between 1984 and 1991 [30]. Bilateral injuries were seen in 42.1% of patients. Acids and alkalis accounted for 80% of chemical ocular injuries in this series. Two-thirds of the injuries occurred in young people working in laboratories and factories. Roper-Hall Grade III and IV injuries were seen in 52 eyes (35.9%). In total, 102 eyes (70.3%) recovered with a visual acuity of 6/60 or better. Ten eyes (6.9%) had no light perception. Phthis bulbi (a deformed eyeball with no light perception) occurred in 71.4% of the seven deliberate chemical assault victims but in only 3.6% of the accidental ocular chemical exposures. The final visual acuity was better in the eyes with less severe grades of chemical injuries on presentation [30].

Cartotto et al. [34] reported a series of patients treated at the burn center in Toronto, Ontario, Canada [34]. Of the total 24 chemical burn cases, there were 8 chemical eye splashes. Five of these eight patients were decontaminated at the scene (presumably with water). The three chemical eye splash patients who did not receive immediate decontamination developed severe ocular injuries. However, three of the five who had immediate decontamination developed corneal erosions and one patient with eye exposure to "black liquor" developed a very deep corneal erosion leading to blindness [34].

Sawheny and Kaudish [35] reported a series of 27 patients with acid and alkali burns treated over a 5-year period in Chandigarh, India [35]. Eye involvement was present in 74% of these patients, with both eyes involved in 15%. Severe conjunctivitis was present in all patients with eye burns, with 63% having keratitis and corneal ulcerations progressing to opacities. Corneal perforation progressing to panophthalmitis and vision loss occurred in two cases. Twelve patients developed severe eyelid ectropion [35].

Mozingo et al. [36] reported a series of 87 chemical burn patients treated at the US Army Institute of Surgical Research from 1969 through 1985 [36]. Associated injuries included chemical eye burns in three patients. In an earlier report from this same institution, the authors noted: "The high incidence of peri-orbital and ocular complications is significant…"

In a retrospective study of patients admitted to the Royal Brisbane Hospital in Australia over a 7-year period, eye burns comprised 5.5% of the total (and included chemical exposures, gas explosions, and electric flashes) [13]. Eye burns were present in 4 (3.7%) patients and eyelid burns were present in 4.6% of patients [13].

2.4 Involved Chemicals

Table 2.1 lists some chemical substances reported to cause ocular chemical injuries.

2.5 Conclusions

Ocular chemical injuries are a significant problem. Existing published data on the epidemiology of such injuries are incomplete. Currently recommended decontamination with water or other commonly available solutions such as normal saline cannot always prevent serious eye injuries. Alternative *active* eye decontamination solutions should continue to be investigated.

Table 2.1 Some chemical substances reported to cause ocular chemical injury

Chemical substance	References
Acids (not further specified)	[28, 30, 35]
Alkalis (not further specified)	[23, 30]
Aluminum hydroxide	[30]
Ammonia	[22, 27]
Ammonium hydroxide	[30]
"Black liquor" (a heated mixture of sodium carbonate, sodium hydroxide, sodium thiosulfate, and sodium sulfate)	[34]
Calcium hydroxide	[30]
Chili powder	[30]
Corrosive substances	[18]
Cracker powder	[30]
Endoxan injection	[30]
Fish bile	[6]
Hydrochloric acid	[30]
Hydrofluoric acid	[30, 33]
Kerosene oil	[30]
Lye	[24, 25]
Methanol	[30]
Nitric acid	[30, 33]
Oxalic acid	[30]
Paint	[30]
Phenol	[30]
Savion	[30]
Sodium hydroxide	[30]
Sulfuric acid	[30]
Unknown	[30]

References

1. Hall, A.H., Maibach, H.I.: Water decontamination of chemical skin/eye splashes: a critical review. Cutaneous Ocular Toxicol **25**, 67–83 (2006)
2. Pfister, R.R.: The effects of chemical injury on the corneal surface. Ophthalmology **90**, 601–609 (1983)
3. Liao, C.-C., Rossignol, A.M.: Landmarks in burn prevention. Burns **26**, 422–434 (2000)
4. Josset, P., Meyer, M.C., Blomet, J.: Pénétration d'un toxique dans le cornée. Etude experimental et simulation [French]. [Penetration of a toxic agent into the cornea. Experimental study and simulation]. SMT **85**, 25–33 (1986)
5. Herr, R.D., White, G.L., Bernhisel, K., Mamalis, N., Swanson, E.: Clinical comparison of ocular irrigation fluids following chemical injury. Am J Emerg Med **9**, 228–231 (1991)
6. Melsaether, C.N., Rosen, C.L.: Burns, Ocular. http://www.emedicine.com, last updated November 1, 2007. Accessed 07/07/2008

References

7. Karaman, K., Gverović-Antunica, A., Rogošić, V., Lakoŝ-Krželj, V., Rozga, A., Rodočaj-Perko, S.: Epidemiology of adult eye injuries in Split-Dalmation County. Croat Med J **45**, 304–309 (2004)
8. Poon, A.S., Ng, J.S., Lam, D.S., Fan, D.S., Leung, A.T.: Epidemiology of severe childhood eye injuries that required hospitalization. Hong Kong Med J **4**, 371–374 (1998)
9. Islam, S.S., Doyle, E.J., Velilla, A., Martin, C.J., Ducatman, A.M.: Epidemiology of compensable work-related ocular injuries and illnesses: incidence and risk factors. J Occup Environ Med **42**, 575–581 (2000)
10. Nicaeus, T., Erb, C., Rohrbach, M., Thiel, H.J.: An analysis of 148 outpatient treated occupational accidents [German]. Klin Monatsbl Augenheilkd **209**, A7–A11 (1996)
11. Kuckelkorn, R., Kottek, A., Schrage, N., Reim, M.: Poor prognosis of severe chemical and thermal eye burns: the need for adequate emergency care and primary prevention. Int Arch Occup Environ Health **67**, 281–284 (1995)
12. Saari, K.M., Parvi, V.: Occupational eye injuries in Finland. Acta Ophthalmol Suppl **161**, 17–28 (1984)
13. Pegg, S.P., Miller, P.M., Sticklen, E.J., Storie, W.J.: Epidemiology of industrial burns in Brisbane. Burns Incl Therm Inj **12**, 484–490 (1986)
14. Moon, M.E., Roberston, I.F.: Retrospective study of alkali burns of the eye. Aust J Ophthalmol **11**, 281–286 (1983)
15. Kersjes, M.P., Reifler, D.M., Maurer, J.R., Trestrail, J.H., McCoy, D.J.: A review of chemical eye burns referred to the Blodgett Regional Poison Center. Vet Hum Toxicol **29**, 453–455 (1987)
16. Bronstein, A.C., Spyker, D.A., Cantilena, L.R., Green, J., Rumack, B.H., Heard, S.E.: 2006 annual report of the American Association of Poison Centers' National Poison Data System (NPDS). Clin Toxicol **45**, 815–917 (2007)
17. Nonfatal occupational injuries and illnesses requiring days away from work, 2006. United States Bureau of Labor, News, Whashington, DC, November 8, 2007. Accessed online in 2008 http://www.bls.gov/iff/home.htm.
18. Hunt, J.P., Calvert, C.T., Peck, M.D., Meyer, A.A.: Occupation-related burn injuries. J Burn Care Rehabil **21**, 327–332 (2000)
19. Kuckelkorn, R., Makropoulos, W., Kottek, A., Reim, M.: Prospective study of severe alkali burns of the eyes [German]. Klin Monatsbl Augenheilkd **203**, 397–402 (1993)
20. Ho, C.K., Yen, Y.L., Chang, C.H., Chiang, H.C., Shen, Y.Y., Chang, P.Y.: Epidemiologic study on work-related eye injuries in Kaohsiung, Taiwan. Kaohsiung J Med Sci **23**, 463–469 (2007)
21. Micheau, P., Lawers, F., Vagth, S.B., Seilha, T., Dumuriger, C., Joly, B.: Caustic burns: Clinical study of 24 patients with sulfuric acid burns in Cambodia [French]. Ann Chir Plast Esthet **49**, 239–254 (2004)
22. Beare, J.D.L.: Eye injuries from assault with chemicals. Br J Ophthalmol **74**, 514–518 (1990)
23. O'Driscoll, A.M., Aggarwal, R.K., Shah, P., Chell, P.B., Hope-Ross, M.W., McDonnell, P.J.: Ocular injuries due to alkaline substances. BMJ **310**, 943 (1995)
24. Yeong, E.K., Chen, M.T., Mann, R., Kin, T.-W., Engrav, L.H.: Facial mutilation after an assault with chemicals: 15 cases and literature review. J Burn Care Rehabil **18**, 234–237 (1997)
25. Crikelair, G.F., Symonds, F.C., Ollstein, R.N., Kirsner, A.I.: Burn causation: its many sides. J Trauma **8**, 572–582 (1968)
26. Faga, A., Scevola, D., Mezzetti, M.G., Scevola, S.: Sulphuric acid burned women in Bangladesh: a social and medical problem. Burns **26**, 701–709 (2000)
27. Merle, H., Donnio, A., Ayeboua, L., Michel, F., Thomas, F., Ketterle, J., et al.: Alkali ocular burns in Martinique (French West Indies): evaluation of the use of an amphoteric solution as the rinsing product. Burns **31**, 670–673 (2005)
28. Branday, J., Arscott, G.D.L., Smoot, E.C., Fletcher, P.R.: Chemical burns as assault injuries in Jamaica. Burns **22**, 154–155 (1996)
29. Asaria, J., Kobusingye, O.C., Khingi, B.A., Balikuddembe, R., Gomez, M., Beveridge, M.: Acid burns from personal assault in Uganda. Burns **30**, 78–81 (2004)
30. Saini, J.S., Sharma, A.: Ocular chemical burns – clinical and demographic profile. Burns **19**, 67–69 (1993)
31. Kaiserman, I., Kaiserman, N.: Severe blepharoconjunctivitis induced by a peeling mask containing trichloroacetic acid. Ocular Immunol Inflamm **13**, 257–259 (2005)
32. Fung, J.F., Sengelmann, R.D., Kenneally, C.Z.: Chemical injury to the eye from trichloroacetic acid. Dermatol Surg **28**, 609–610 (2002)
33. Xie, Y., Tan, Y., Tang, S.: Epidemiology of 377 patients with chemical burns in Guangdong province. Burns **30**, 569–572 (2004)
34. Cartotto, R.C., Peters, W.J., Neligan, P.C., Douglas, L.G., Beeston, J.: Chemical burns. Can J Surg **39**, 205–211 (1996)
35. Sawheny, C.P., Kaudish, R.: Acid and alkali burns: considerations in management. Burns **15**, 132–134 (1989)
36. Mozingo, D.W., Smith, A.A., McManus, W.F., Pruitt, B.A., Mason, A.D.: Chemical burns. J Trauma **26**, 642–647 (1988)
37. Milton, R., Mathieu, L., Hall, A.H., Maibach, H.I.: Chemical assault and skin/eye burns: two representative cases, report from the Acid Survivors Foundation, and literature review. Burns **36**, 924–32 (2010)

The Chemical Agents and the Involved Chemical Reactions

François Burgher, Laurence Mathieu, and Joël Blomet

3.1 From Chemistry to Symptoms

3.1.1 What Is a Chemical Burn?

The ocular chemical burn is the result of the destruction of a more or less important quantity of biochemical constituents of the cells of living tissues when in contact with an irritant or corrosive chemical.

Corrosives and irritants are mainly acids, bases, oxidizing agents, reductors, chelators, alkylating agents, and solvents.

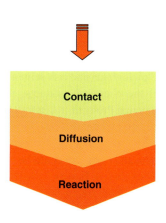

Fig. 3.1 Parameters affecting the chemical burn

3.1.2 What Are the Parameters Affecting the Chemical Burn?

The first damages to tissues do not develop within the first seconds of contact with a corrosive. They progressively and quickly take place only when the penetration phase starts from the surface of the cornea toward the deeper layers.

The seriousness of a chemical burn depends on (Fig. 3.1):

- The nature and concentration of the chemical
- The energetic level of the chemical reaction
- The length of contact
- The physical characteristics of the chemical (solid, viscous, etc.) or the specific conditions of use (under high pressure, at hot temperature, etc.)

3.1.3 Extent of the Matter

Chemicals are omnipresent in our world today. Chemical risk is a permanent issue in our everyday environment, obviously on work premises, and may also be caused by different circumstances of chemical assaults. Among all chemical accidents, eye projections are a specific issue because of the vulnerability of ocular structures and also because of the risk of major functional after-effects. Chemical Abstracts Service (CAS) is a division of the American Chemical Society. This International database of the American Chemical Society is a worldwide reference registering

F. Burgher (✉), L. Mathieu, and J. Blomet
PREVOR Laboratory, Moulin de Verville,
95760 Valmondois, France
e-mail: fburgher@prevor.com;
lmathieu@prevor.com;
jblomet@prevor.com

most of the existing molecules – including organic and inorganic. In April 2010 the CAS registered, in all, more than 61 million substances. Among these, more than 25,000 irritant and corrosive chemicals were identified as having the potential to cause burns [1].

In Europe, 100,204 commercial chemical substances have been recognized and numbered under EINECS (European INventory of Existing Commercial chemical Substances) by the European Chemical Bureau (ECB) System. Another 4,381 "new" substances are classified under ELINCS Information System (European LIst of Notified Chemical Substances) since May 11, 1981. Among these, In Europe 1,230 chemical substances are officially identified as irritant or corrosive with Xi and C pictograms and risk sentences.

Among all the chemical products, the American EPA (Environmental Protection Agency) has estimated that there are approximately 100,000 chemicals in commercial use in the USA. So the same amount of identified irritant and corrosive could be expected to be found in the USA than in Europe.

Considering the high frequency of potential chemical risk and the wide diversity of the substances that might be involved, it is important to better understand the deep mechanisms of the chemical reactivity of irritants and corrosives on the eye. This will help to optimize the management of eye chemical projections. Besides, we have learned by experience that the rapidity and efficiency of the emergency decontamination are decisive parameters in order to prevent the development of potentially severe lesions and after-effects due to the chemical eye burn.

We will develop the following points:

1. The chemical agent, its nature, and the intensity of its reactivity
2. The mechanisms of the chemical burn during the contact between the aggressor and the eye
3. The practical conclusions for an optimal management of the eye chemical decontamination

3.2 The Chemical Agent

The chemical agent is made of a molecular skeleton on which are connected some functional groups responsible for the expression of various kinds of reactivity. The presence of modulator groups enables to vary the intensity of this reactivity according to electronic rules involving either simple connections bonds (inductive effect) or double connections bonds (mesomeric effect).

Six elementary types of chemical reactivity are listed as follows:

- Acid–base reaction
- Reduction/oxidation (or redox)
- Chelation
- Addition
- Substitution
- Solvation

From a fundamental point of view, the strength of each of these reactions can be conceptualized on a scale of energy. This scale is defined by the reactional Δg, which is the free enthalpy.

This one, in practice, can be specifically declined for every type of elementary reactivity:

- The pK scale for acid–base reactions
- The potential scale for oxidants and reducing agents
- The complexation constant for chelating agents
- ΔG (the Gibbs function = reactional energy) for alkylating agents
- Partition coefficient for solvents

The energy scale is based on the notion of strength and weakness. There is a specific scale for each kind of reactivity. It is then essential to study what makes a molecule active or not and what are the parameters influencing the strength of reactivity of a molecule. The fine distinction between an irritant and a corrosive substance appeals to this principle of scale and energy level. The strength of reactivity directly conditions the speed of appearance of the reaction of the tissues, the constitution of more or less important lesions, and their more or less irreversible characteristics. We can so connect the chemical reactivity and the severity of the chemical burn lesions.

3.2.1 Molecular Structure of an Irritant or a Corrosive

Literally, a molecule is a compound of atoms connected to each other by various kinds of bonds.

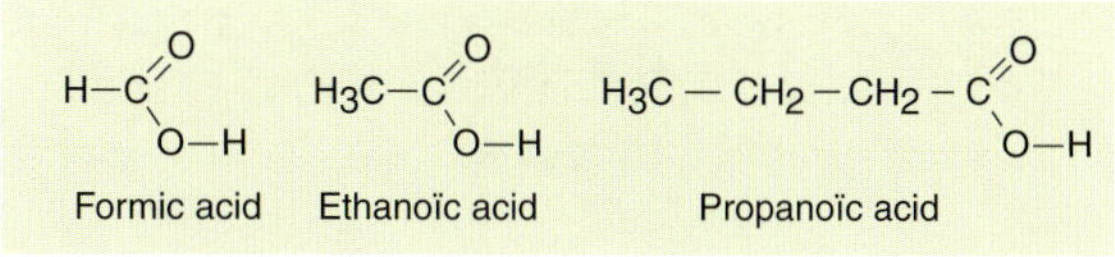

3.2 The Chemical Agent

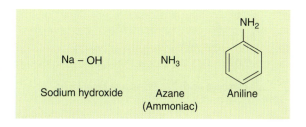

Fig. 3.2 Organic structure of corrosive agents

An irritant or a corrosive agent is, most of the times:

- A simple mineral entity: HCl, HF, HNO$_3$, H$_2$O$_2$, H$_2$SO$_4$, NaOH, KOH, etc.
- An organic structure with a low molecular weight, based on a carbonated structure, for instance, formic acid, acetic acid, or propanoic acid (Fig. 3.2), etc.

Thus, the irritant and corrosive agents can be easily considered as molecular entities. In most cases, they are small or even very small structures (like hydrofluoric acid – HF, for instance).

3.2.2 Reactive Functional Groups of Irritant or Corrosive Agents

In a simplistic vision, molecular structures have one or, more scarcely, several functional groups. These groups, of diverse nature, provide the expression of the reactivity of a molecule. They are functions such as:

3.2.2.1 Acidic Function

H$^+$ results either from mineral acids or from carboxylic acids (–COOH function) or from alcohol function (–OH) or thiol function (–SH) (Fig. 3.3).

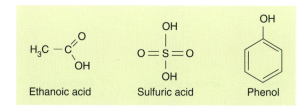

Fig. 3.3 Examples of acidic molecules

Fig. 3.4 Examples of basic molecules

3.2.2.2 Basic Function

The basic function defines the substances called bases. Either mineral or organic, these substances have the following properties:

- To release an OH$^-$ ion
- The ability to capture a proton (H$^+$ ion), for instance, an amine group (–NH$_2$), or a function including a triple bond: ≡N (Fig. 3.4)

Energy Scale of Acid–Base Reactions: The pK Notion

When an acid dissolves in water, a certain proportion of the molecule dissociates:

$$AH \rightarrow A^- + H^+$$

For any given molecule, the dissociated fraction in water is always equal. It is an intrinsic property of the molecule in relation with the connection forces between its constitutive atoms in water.

This constant is called K_a. The bigger the K_a constant, the bigger the dissociated fraction and the stronger the acidity.

$$K_a = [A^-] \times [H^+]/[AH]$$

The same reasoning works for the dissociation of bases with a constant of basicity called K_b. To make things easier, it is the logarithmic value of K, called pK, that is commonly used: $pK_a = -\log_{10} K_a$.

3.2.2.3 Oxidizing Function

Some reagents can capture one or several electrons and be part of an oxidation reaction. They are called

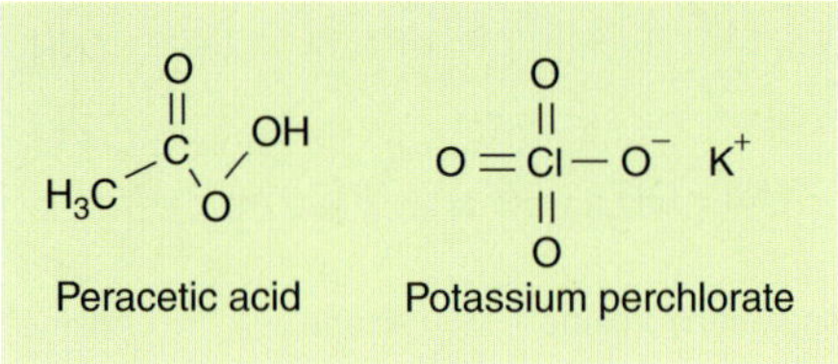

Fig. 3.5 Examples of oxidizing function

oxidizers. They are either mineral, like $KMnO_4$ or CrO_3, or organic, like peracids (Fig. 3.5).

3.2.2.4 Reduction Function

Some reagents can release one or several electrons and be part of a reduction reaction. They are called reducing agents. Reducing agents are mineral, like Li, Na, or $AlLiH_4$, or organic, like hydrazine (Fig. 3.6).

The redox potential is the energy scale of the redox reaction. It evaluates the importance of the oxidizing or the reducing property. Pure water is taken as a reference. Therefore, the value of the redox couple of water is said to be zero.

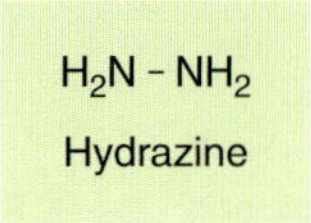

Fig. 3.6 Example of reduction function

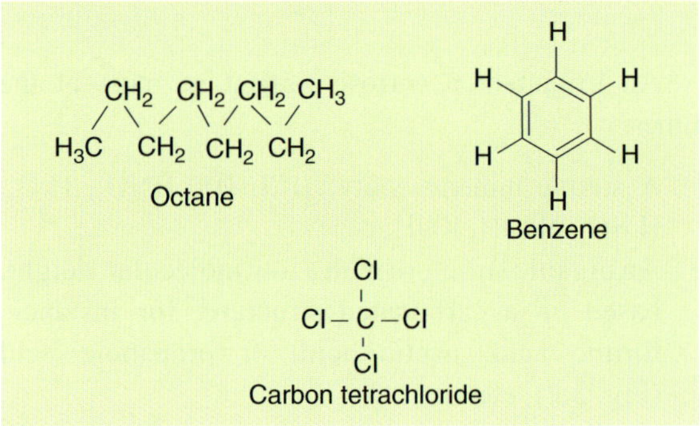

Fig. 3.7 Examples of apolar solvents

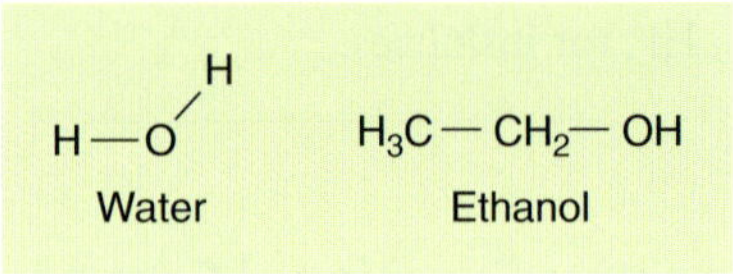

Fig. 3.8 Examples of protic polar solvents

3.2.2.5 Solvent Function

The solvation expresses according to a set of physico-chemical characteristics. We distinguish several big families of solvents with varied structures or varied functional groups [6]:

- *Apolar solvents*, hydrocarbonated structure that are electronically symmetric molecules (Fig. 3.7).
- *Protic polar solvents*, like water – omnipresent in the body – or functions such as alcohol (–OH) or thiol (–SH) (Fig. 3.8). A molecule is said to be protic when it can release a proton. The connection between the hydrogen and another atom is weak enough. A molecule that cannot release a proton is called aprotic. A molecule is said to be polar when, without any electronic field, the center of gravity of the negative charges is different from the center of gravity of the positive charges.
- *Aprotic polar solvents*, with functions such as ketone (>C=O), nitrile (–CN), amide (O=C–NH$_2$), sulfoxide (>S=O), ether (–O–), and halogenated and electronically asymmetric solvents (Figs. 3.9 and 3.10).

The partition coefficient of solvents is also a reactional energy scale.

A substance has more or less of affinity and it thus dissolves more easily in a type of solvent than in the other one. We call partition coefficient the constant

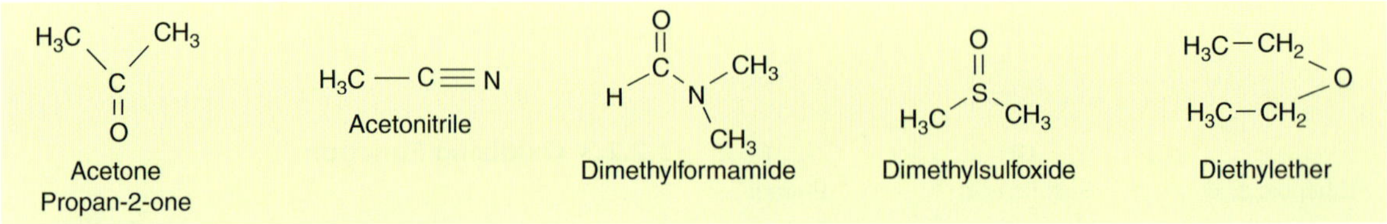

Fig. 3.9 Examples of aprotic polar solvents

3.2 The Chemical Agent

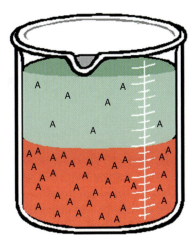

Fig. 3.10 Trichloroethane

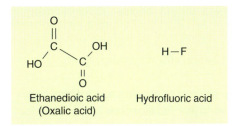

$K_{o/w} = 7/33$

Fig. 3.11 Solvent's partition coefficient

Chemical	Log P value
Acetamide	−1.16
Methanol	−0.82
Ethyl acetate	−0.68
Formic acid	−0.41
Ethanol	−0.28
Diethylether	0.83
1-Pentanol	1.39
Phenol	1.42
Nitrobenzene	1.84
Benzene	2.14
Chlororbenzene	2.80
Bromobenzene	2.99
p-Dichlorobenzene	3.37
Hexamethylbenzene	4.61
Pentachlorobenzene	4.99

Fig. 3.12 Values of some partition coefficients

Fig. 3.13 Chelator agents (Ethanedioic acid (Oxalic acid), Hydrofluoric acid)

that measures the proportion of the substance within each of both phases proposed. In common practice we use water (as phase of aqueous nature) and octanol (as phase of lipidic type) (Fig. 3.11).

Therefore, the partition coefficient enables to foresee with figures the behavior of a given substance (the solute) in a hydrophilic or lipophilic solvent environment. Some examples of partition coefficients are given in Fig. 3.12.

3.2.2.6 Chelating Function or Complexation

Chelation (literally pliers or pincers) is the formation of a complex made of a chelating agent, a ligand, and a cation or a metallic atom that is set in the center of the complex. The atom or cation is connected by at least two connections called coordination bonds. Illustrations of important chelating reactions found in ocular corrosive damages: the calcium and magnesium ions with oxalic acid or with the fluor ion of hydrofluoric acid (Fig. 3.13).

Energy Scale of Chelation Reactions

The molecular complexation constant expresses the strength of the bond. A weak chelation results in an unsteady and labile complex. A high constant results in a very stable compound that will not tend to dissociate.

3.2.2.7 Alkylation Reaction

The notion of alkylation is linked to the concept of adduct and therefore to the mechanism of addition of a substrate to another one. An adduct is a piece of chemical covalently bonded to another molecule. If the adduct concern DNA, it can cause carcinogenesis.

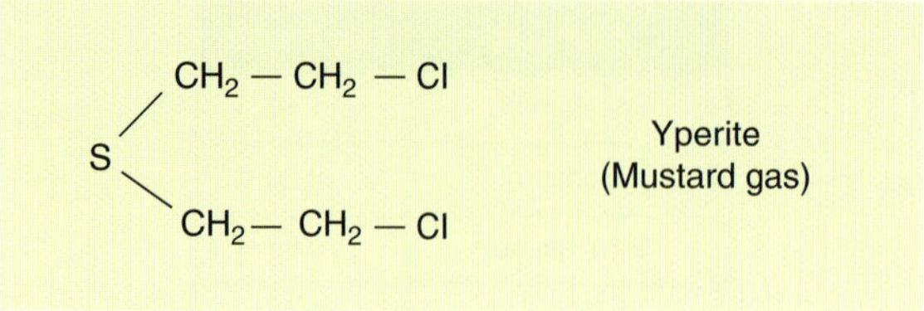

```
         CH₂ — CH₂ — Cl
       /
     S                          Yperite
       \                      (Mustard gas)
         CH₂ — CH₂ — Cl
```

Fig. 3.14 Yperite (mustard gas)

But alkylation can also involve a mechanism of substitution. More accurately, this will appeal to the electrophilia-neutrophilia couple, and therefore to the ΔG scale with a substrate lacking electrons and eager to settle on an electron-rich part of molecule, for instance an amine group (NH$_2$), or oxygen, nitrogen, or sulfur atoms.

To be compared with the reaction on residue of amino acids of human proteins.

The result of an alkylation gives way to the connection of a carbon chain of variable size with another molecular structure. In matter of corrosiveness, alkylation (particularly when happening on the proteins of ocular tissues) may cause severe burns. A historical example is given by a war gas such as yperite or mustard gas (Fig. 3.14). Other alkylating molecules are used in anticarcinogenic chemotherapies.

Reactivity Scale for Alkylating Agents

After a reaction of alkylation, a balance settles within the system. The balance constant is a thermodynamic value. In matter of energy, this situation is called free enthalpy or Gibbs free energy.

3.2.2.8 Molecular Reactivity and Chemical Bonds: Main Aspects

The relative fragility of the connections between the constitutive atoms of the molecule is an intrinsic property of the structure. This strength of connection is conditioned by the properties of the constitutive atoms. The breaking of the intramolecular chemical connections enables the release of atoms, ions, or groups of atoms that have the ability to exchange with other molecular entities.

For instance, acetic acid is acid because, when its O–H bond breaks, the CH$_3$COOH molecule can release an H$^+$ ion (or proton), which is the cause of the acidity (Fig. 3.15).

$$CH_3COOH \longrightarrow CH_3COO^- + H^+$$

Fig. 3.15 Acetic acid

$$TiCl_4 + 4H_2O \longrightarrow Ti(OH)_4 + 4HCl$$

Fig. 3.16 Titanium salts

$$BF_3 + 3H_2O \longrightarrow B(OH)_3 + 3HF$$

Fig. 3.17 Boron trifluoride

There are also chemicals that can generate corrosive or irritant agents, when reacting with other species such as water. They could be called pro-irritant or pro-corrosive agents. For instance, it is the case of titanium's salts (See Sect. 3.4.3.1, Figs. 3.65), bore, silane, alkyl aluminium, isocyanates, or Lewis acid (Figs. 3.16 and 3.17).

3.2.3 Modulation of the Expression of the Reactivity of a Molecule

The presence of atoms or groups of atoms, called "modulators," close to the reactional group as described above, in the molecular structure explains the variation of the intensity of the reactional expression.

We will show this for five different ocular corrosives:

- Acetic acid and its derivatives
- Hydrofluoric acid
- Phenol
- Methylamines
- Acrolein

3.2.3.1 Acetic Acid and Its Derivatives

Acetic acid of vinegar is commonly known as a weak acid. This is a consequence of the relative strength of the bond between the hydrogen and oxygen atoms as parts of the –OH group in the –COOH carboxylic function (Fig. 3.18).

3.2 The Chemical Agent

![Acetic acid dissociation figure]

Fig. 3.18 Acetic acid dissociation

Fig. 3.21 Hydrofluoric acid

The worst ocular damage caused by a drop of vinegar might be a harmless irritation.

When the second carbon atom of the structure is bonded with one, two, or three chlorine atoms, the electronic sharing of the whole molecule is modified and its acidity increases (Fig. 3.19). This effect of modulation is the result of the chlorine atoms being, as the other halogens, electro attractive for the electronic doublet bonding them with a carbon atom. If this doublet moves toward the center of the chlorine atom, a part of it is taken away from the connected carbon atom. This one will then automatically try to compensate this loss by attracting its other bonding doublets, and particularly the one shared with the oxygen atom from the hydroxyl group (–OH) of the acid function. This misbalance of electronic charges will weaken the O–H bond. It is then easy to understand that the hydrogen atom, less strongly connected, will release more easily as an H^+ ion. Then the acidic characteristic is more outstanding. The addition of a second and a third chlorine atom will amplify this effect (Fig. 3.19).

As shown in the table below (Fig. 3.20), acidity gets stronger as acetic acid changes to trichloroacetic acid, which is a major corrosive and a very damaging acid. More chlorine atoms mean more acidity.

3.2.3.2 Hydrofluoric Acid

The same type of mechanism happens with a molecule of hydrofluoric acid. The very strong electro negativity of fluor attracts a part of the electronic cloud of the hydrogen atom (Fig. 3.21). A strong polarization of the molecule happens because of the concentration of negativity (δ^-) on the side of the fluor atom center, and the opposing δ^+ generated by the loss of a part of the electronic cloud on the hydrogen side.

Such a misbalance weakens the bond H–F so much that, in water, the fluor atom will definitely capture the electron originally coming from the hydrogen atom. The fluor atom will then turn into a F^- ion. Because of losing its unique electron, the hydrogen atom becomes an H^+ ion. Combining the acidity of the hydrogen ion, and mostly the toxicity of the fluor ion, the resulting dissociated molecule is highly corrosive. We will study the consequences of HF eye burns in Sect. 3.4.1 (Fig. 3.57).

3.2.3.3 Phenol

The phenol molecule is another illustration of modulation. Its name ending with the suffix -ol and its hydroxyl function (–OH) define it as an alcohol. But, it is a weak

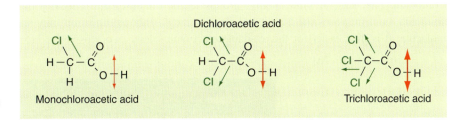

Fig. 3.19 Chlorinated acetic acids dissociation

Acids	Formula	PK$_a$
Acetic	CH$_3$–COOH	4.76
Monochloracetic	ClCH$_2$–COOH	2.87
Dichloracetic	Cl$_2$CH–COOH	1.25
Trichloroacetic	Cl$_3$C–COOH	0.66

Fig. 3.20 pK of acetic acid chlorinated derivatives

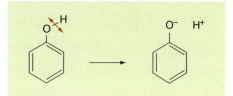

Fig. 3.22 Phenol

acid too (pK = 9.3), because, thanks to the weakness of its O–H bond, the phenol molecule can release an H+ ion. In such a case, the doublet bonding the oxygen and carbon atoms moves toward the aromatic cycle that acts as an electron attractor (Fig. 3.22).

This acidic characteristic may be only slightly outstanding indeed. But a high concentration of phenol can generate severe corrosion lesions. Once again, the toxicity of the phenolate ion completes the deletery mechanism of destruction of the ocular tissues.

3.2.3.4 Methylamines Series

This is another example illustrating the modulation of the basal expression of the NH_2 group according to the growing number of substituting groups. We have studied above the electro attractive properties of halogens and aromatic cycle. On the opposite, some modulators are called electro-donors. They cause a contrary effect of stabilization of the bonds and reinforce the electronic cloud of the atom they are bonded with. These electro-donor modulator groups are alkyl chains (methyl –CH_3, ethyl CH_3–CH_2–, propyl CH_3–CH_2–CH_2–, etc.). Combining one, two, or three methyl groups to the ammonia atom increases the basicity of the resulting molecule. It is then easier for the available electronic

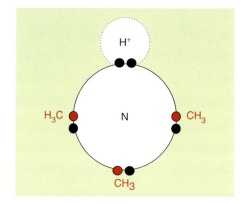

Fig. 3.23 Trimethylamine

doublet to receive an H+ ion (per say a hydrogen with an empty orbital) (Fig. 3.23).

The capture of H+ ions from the chemical environment modifies the original H+/OH− balance of water and increases the proportion of OH− ions. Therefore, the solution becomes basic and this basicity is the cause of the general irritant characteristic of the aliphatic amines.

This effect is maximal for dimethylamine. It is less important with trimethylamine because of the steric saturation and of its solvation limiting the inductive effect (Fig. 3.24).

3.2.3.5 Last Illustration: Acrolein

In an aromatic cycle or in an unsaturated carbon chain, the doublets Π of the double bonds may move and thus modify the reactivity of the molecule. For instance, this modification may specifically happen with acrolein – a corrosive (and toxic) molecule (Fig. 3.25):

Base	Formula	PK$_a$	PK$_b$
Ammonia	NH_3	9.25	4.75
Methylamine	CH_3–NH_2	10.66	3.34
Dimethylamine	$(CH_3)_2$–NH	10.73	3.27
Trimethylamine	$(CH_3)_3$–N	9.80	4.2

Fig. 3.24 pK values of methyl derivatives

3.2 The Chemical Agent

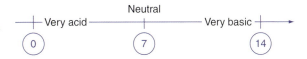

Fig. 3.25 Acrolein

This is called the mesomeric effect. The move of electronic doublets due to the mesomeric effect generates charges on the carbon and oxygen atoms of acrolein.

Therefore, there are two different effects applying to the structure of a molecule:

- Inductive effects implying the doublet acting in a simple bond linking two atoms.
- Mesomeric effects implying the doublets acting in the double bonds linking two atoms.

3.2.4 Energetic Levels of the Chemical Reactivity

It is easily understood by intuition that acids, bases, oxidants, chelators, etc. express their reactivity with more or less intensity. Some are called a strong acid, a weak oxidant. In Sect. 3.4.3.1, we will study the importance of the applications of this theoretical approach for the understanding and the prediction of the importance of ocular lesions in case of corrosive projections.

What are these notions of levels of reactivity and what are the scales we can use to evaluate these?

3.2.4.1 Acid–Base Scale

In general, the strength of an acid is measured by its capacity to release H^+ ions in water. Other liquids can be used instead of water, like ammonia. We then define an acid–base couple, using the example of hydrochloric acid in aqueous environment (Fig. 3.26).

Strong acids spontaneously and completely dissociate in water and thus release all their acidity. The notion of pH shows up the notion of strong acidity or basicity, as related in the following relation (Fig. 3.27).

The pH value is very important for chemistry as well as for biology (Fig. 3.28).

In usual conditions, the pH of blood is 7.35, the pH of saliva is 7, and the pH of tears slightly varies from 6.9 to 7.5. When the pH is different from these values, a feeling of pain and an effect of irritation or even corrosion will appear.

For an acid–base couple, the relation is (Fig. 3.29):

This allows the definition of the acidity constant of the reaction (Fig. 3.30):

By analogy with the pH, we consider $pK_a = -\log K_a$.

Therefore, the pH relation is (Fig. 3.31).

The stronger the AH acid is and more the balance of the reaction moves into the direct way, the bigger the K_a constant and the smaller the pK value.

We can then deduce (Fig. 3.32).

Therefore, for a solution with a given pH, the predominance of species of the acid–base couple can be stated as follows (Fig. 3.33).

Fig. 3.26 Acido–basic reaction

$$pH = -\log [H^+] \text{ for a strong acid}$$
$$\text{and}$$
$$pH = 14 + \log [H^+] \text{ for a strong base}$$

Fig. 3.27 pH

Fig. 3.28 pH scale

$$A-H \longrightarrow A^- + H^+$$

Fig. 3.29 Acido–basic couple

$$K_a = [A^-] \times [H^+] / [AH]$$

Fig. 3.30 Acid dissociation constant

$$pH = pk_a + \log [A^-] / [AH] \text{ or } \log [base] / [acid]$$

Fig. 3.31 pH and pK

[A⁻] = [AH]   pH = pKa

[A⁻] > [AH]   pH > pKa

[A⁻] < [AH]   pH < pKa

Fig. 3.32 pH and pK value comparison

```
                pKa                    pH
────────────────┼──────────────────────►
[AH >> A⁻]   [AH = A⁻]      [AH << A⁻]
```

Fig. 3.33 Predominance of species in acido–basic couple

```
 pK₁ = 2.1      pK₂ = 7.2       pK₃ = 12
─────┼──────────────┼────────────────┼──── pH
H₃PO₄    H₂PO₄⁻         HPO₄²⁻         PO₄³⁻
```

Fig. 3.34 pK values for phosphoric acid

Modifying the pH by one unit up or down on a logarithmic scale is equivalent to a variation of the base/acid concentrations ratio by factor 10 up or down.

Let's illustrate this with phosphoric acid, which is a triacid because of its capacity to successively release 3H⁺ ions one by one. Depending on its pH, it has different shapes (Fig. 3.34):

For instance, with a pH of 8, it is mostly constituted of the HPO₄²⁻ species.

When put together, an acid can react to all the bases set on its right of the scale (Fig. 3.35):

If not dissociating completely in water, an acid is called weak.

In such a case, some of the non-dissociated AH acid molecules remains in water (Fig. 3.36).

The less an acid dissociates, the bigger its pK value and the weaker the acid. It is then less acidic and less harmful to the eye.

The pK scale renders an accurate classification with figures of the strength of acids.

$$A'H \longrightarrow A'H + A'^- + H^+$$

Fig. 3.36 Weak acid in water

$$A^- + H_2O \longrightarrow AH + OH^-$$

Fig. 3.37 Constant of balance of a base with water

$$K_b = \frac{[AH] \times [OH^-]}{[A^-]}$$

Fig. 3.38 Kb equation

And the K_b basicity constant of an acid base AH/A⁻ couple is defined as the constant of balance of the A⁻ base with water (Fig. 3.37).

Therefore, (Fig. 3.38)

The stronger the A⁻ base is and more the balance of the reaction moves into the direct way, the bigger the K_b constant and the smaller the pK_b value, with $pK_b = -\log K_b$ (Fig. 3.39). Strong acids or strong bases exist in water in a dissociated form.

For a weak acid or a weak base, the pH will be calculated according to the pKa by using the following formula: Weak acid solution (Fig. 3.40)

Weak base solution (Fig. 3.41):

Thus, for a 0.1N hydrofluoric acid solution (with $pK_a = 3.2$), the pH calculation relation is (Fig. 3.42):

A solution is said molar if it contains 1 mol, that is, 6.02 10²³ molecules of substance per liter of solution (1M). A molar solution of a monoacid is said Normal (1N). But when an acid or a base is able to liberate more than one acidity (x) or one basicity (y), the solution becomes xN or yN. Practically, the sulfuric acid H₂SO₄ can liberate successively two H⁺. A 1M solution of this acid will be a 2N solution.

For a 1N ammonia solution (with pKa = 9.2), the pH calculation relation is (Fig. 3.43):

Given that from zero and below, completely dissociated acids are said strong acids. This implies the following formula (Fig. 3.44):

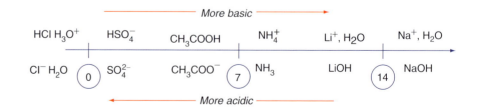

Fig. 3.35 Acid and base reactions

3.2 The Chemical Agent

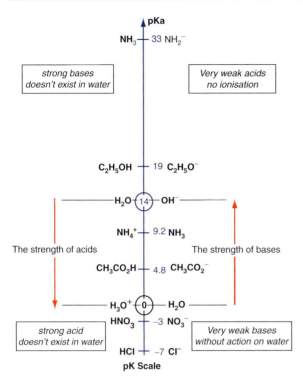

Fig. 3.39 Chemical reactivity of aqueous solutions

$$pH = 1/2\,(pK_a - \log C)$$

With C for Concentration of the acid or base.

Fig. 3.40 pH of a weak acid

$$pH = 7 + 1/2\,(pK_a + \log C)$$

Fig. 3.41 pH of a weak base

$$pH = 1/2\,(pK_a - \log C) = 1/2\,(3.2 - \log 0.1)$$
$$= 1/2\,(3.2 + 1) = 2.1$$

Fig. 3.42 pH of HF in a water solution

$$pH = 7 + 1/2\,(pK_a + \log C) = 7 + 1/2\,(9.2 + 0) = 11.6$$

Fig. 3.43 pH of 1N ammonia solution

$$pH = -\log [C] \text{ for a strong acid}$$
and
$$pH = 14 + \log [C] \text{ for a strong base}$$

Fig. 3.44 pH of strong acid and base

In the following table, we shall find examples of acids, which illustrate, using the pKa value, their more or less important strength (Fig. 3.45).

3.2.4.2 Prediction of the Irritant Power of Acids or Bases

Given the concentration and the pK of the involved corrosive substance, it is possible to predict if a solution of an acid or basic chemical is not aggressive or can be irritant or corrosive to the eye. So we define the notion of threshold concentration as developed below in Sect. 3.4.3.2.

The intermediate zone of the scale – pK between 5 and 9 – is considered as having no aggressive effect for the physiological balance of the cornea. Out of this zone, we can notice either an irritation when the substance is diluted or corrosion when the substance is concentrated.

Below 0.2N, there is no reaction of the tissues. In the intermediate cases, either with a limit pK in the intervals 5–4 and 9–10 or for weakly concentrated solutions (from 0.2 to 1N), there is only an irritation. Only the solutions with a pK lower than 4 or superior to 10 and a concentration of 1N or more are corrosive (Fig. 3.46).

3.2.4.3 Scales of Energy Level

It is easy to understand that every type of reactive chemical function causing an irritation or a corrosion corresponds to a type of elementary reaction (Sect. 3.2).

The intensity of reaction of the chemical aggressor can be represented on a scale of energy, the functioning of which is governed by a simple rule.

- *Thus, in an acid–base solution*, there is an exchange of protons and the relation is (Fig. 3.47). The reaction develops until equilibrium reaching a specific pH. Acid$_1$ reacts on base$_2$ when $pK_1 < pK_2$. The reaction will move even more to the right side when $pK_1 - pK_2$ is big.
- *For oxidizing and reducing agents*, the intrinsic potential E°, measured in volts (V) or millivolts (mV), is the expression of their reactivity and the general rule to apply is: "An oxidizing agent oxidizes every reducing agent with a weaker potential than its own."

The applicable relation is (Fig. 3.48)

Acid	Buffering base	pK_a	Acid	Buffering base	pK_a
HI (the strongest) Hydriodic acid	I^-	−5.2	HOOC–CH$_2$–COOH Malonic acid	HOOC–CH$_2$–COO$^-$	2.9
H$_2$SO$_4$ Sulfuric acid	HSO$_4^-$	−5.0	HF Hydrofluoric acid	F$^-$	3.2
HBr Hydrobromic acid	Br$^-$	−4.7	HOOC–CH=CH–COOH Malic acid	HOOC–CH=CH–COO$^-$	3.4
HCl Hydrochloric acid	Cl$^-$	−2.2	HCOOH Formic acid	HCOO$^-$	3.8
H$_3$O$^+$ Hydronium ion	H$_2$O	0	H$_2$C=CH–COOH Acrylic acid	H$_2$C=OH-COO$^-$	4.25
CH$_3$SO$_3$H Methanesulfonic acid	CH$_3$SO$_3^-$	−1.2	CH$_3$COOH Acetic acid	CH$_3$COO$^-$	4.76
HClO$_3$ Chloric acid	HClO$_3^-$	0	HCN Hydrocyanic acid	CN$^-$	9.2
Cl$_3$C–COOH Trichloroacetic acid	Cl$_3$C–COO$^-$	0.66	C$_6$H$_5$–OH Phenol	C$_6$H$_5$-O$^-$	9.9
H$_2$CrO$_4$ Chromic acid	HCrO$_4^-$	0.8	CH$_3$SH Methanethiol	CH$_3$S$^-$	10.0
H$_2$N–SO$_2$–OH Sulfamic acid	H$_2$N–SO$_2$O$^-$	1.0	CH$_3$OH Methanol	CH$_3$O$^-$	15.5
HOOC–COOH Oxalic acid	HOOC–COO$^-$	1.2	H$_2$O Water	HO$^-$	14
HOOC–CH=CH–COOH Maleic acid	HOOC–CH=CH–COO$^-$	2.0	NH$_3$ Ammonia	H$_2$N$^-$	35
ClCH$_2$–COOH Dichloroacetic acid	ClCH$_2$–COOH	2.87	H$_2$ (the weakest)	H$^-$	38

Fig. 3.45 Acid strength and pK value

3.3 Constituents of the Tissues: Which Are the Biological and Biochemical Targets?

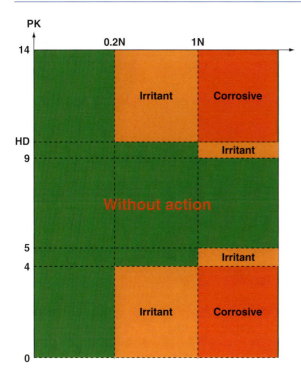

Fig. 3.46 pK, normality, and corrosivity

$$Acid_1 + Base_2 \longleftrightarrow Base_1 + Acid_2$$

Fig. 3.47 Acido–basic solution

$$u_1\, Ox_1 + u_2\, Red_2 \longrightarrow u_1\, Red_1 + u_2\, Ox_2$$

Fig. 3.48 Reaction for oxidizing and reducing agents

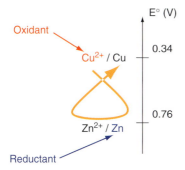

Fig. 3.49 Copper sulfate solution

The reaction develops from left to right when $E°_1 > E°_2$. A good illustration of this rule is a blade of zinc covered with lead, disaggregated and oxidized in a copper sulfate solution (Fig. 3.49).

$$R\!-\!O\!-\!H \longrightarrow RO^- + H^+$$
$$H^+ + Base^- \longrightarrow BH$$

Fig. 3.50 Acidic potential of an alcohol

- *For chelating agents*, we will use the complexation constant.
- *For addition and substitution*, it will be the electrophilic/nucleophilic character.
- *For solvents*, finally, it will be a combination of physical parameters such as the partition coefficient coupled with the potential of chemical reactivity. For example, it is easy to understand that, for alcohols, this chemical potential may be relative to a certain degree of acidity due to the possible break of the connection between the hydrogen atom and the oxygen atom, when the molecule is in a basic environment (Fig. 3.50).

For solvents, the value of this constant is expressed in logarithmic unit for the same practical reasons as for the acid–base scale:

$$\log P = \log K_{o/w}$$

It is the differential measurement of the solubility of a product in two solvents (with O figuring octanol and W figuring water). When log P is very high, the chemical compound under study reveals much more soluble in octanol than in water. Therefore, the chemical compound has a much more lipophilic character. Conversely, when log P is low, the chemical substance is more hydrophilic. When log P equals zero, the chemical is equally split in two solvent phases.

Therefore, the partition coefficient (log P) enables to foresee with figures the behavior of a given substance (the solute) in a hydrophilic or lipophilic solvent environment.

A further step can be reached by linking log P with pH and pKa: log D is a measure of log P for a certain pH value with a product having a pK value.

$$\log D = \log P - [1 + 10^{(pH-pKa)}].$$

3.3 Constituents of the Tissues: Which Are the Biological and Biochemical Targets?

As an organ, the eye is constituted by various structures each formed by a specifically differentiated cellular tissue: the transparent cornea, the aqueous humor of the anterior chamber, the lamellar lens, etc. Each of these structures is constituted by a large number of cells. Every cell presents substructures concentrating one very large number of assemblies of more or less complex molecules.

The histological description is to be studied in Chap. 4 and anatomy in Chap. 7.

But, for us, everything is naturally molecular chemistry in an ultrastructural scale. This mechanistic and materialistic approach might surprise any doctor? Nevertheless not only this molecular organization of the living substance is real but it even helps to understand the intimacy of the eye chemical danger and the ultimate consequences of chemical burns.

The living substance is constituted by six major atomic elements entering the architecture of the biochemical molecules. They are carbon, which defines the organic chemistry (that is the chemistry of what's alive), hydrogen, oxygen, nitrogen, phosphorus, and sulfur. It is necessary to add to these five other elements of mainly ionic nature included in trace elements: Na (Na$^+$), Mg (Mg^{++}), K (K$^+$), Ca (Ca^{++}), Cl (Cl$^-$). These ions are essential to keep the balance of aqueous biological environments whether they are in intra- or extracellular environments.

The three kinds of biological substrates are results of the combination of these elements:

- *Lipids* are mostly more or less long hydrocarbon chain molecules, constituting particularly the cell membranes and the mitochondria membrane (Figs. 3.51 and 3.52).
- *Glucides or carbohydrates* combine carbon, hydrogen, and oxygen (carbohydrates) inside isolated molecular structures, gathered in macromolecules (glycogen) or connected to proteins (glycoproteins). Figure 3.53 illustrates the example of a sugar: glucose.
- *Proteins* may have a gigantic size and are constituted of the chaining of tens to several hundred various amino acids. They contribute to the support of the cell structural architecture, to the transport of numerous compounds by blood and most of all they have enzymatic properties of catalysis of biochemical reactions (Fig. 3.54).

As studied above, chemical burns are always the result of an elementary chemical reaction during the contact of two entities, one "the aggressor," the other

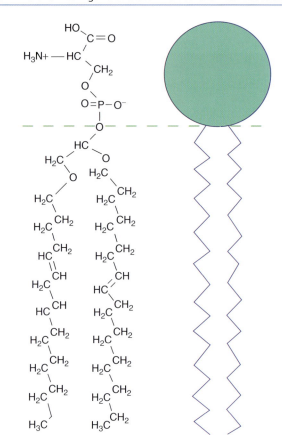

Fig. 3.51 Phospholipid chemical structure

one "the assaulted," in chemistry, the reagent and the reactant.

We understand easily that the corrosive chemical agents can give very quickly a fatal blow to the cells constituting organic tissues of organs, in different ways:

- Damaging cytoplasmic membranes
- Disintegrating the three-dimensional configuration of proteins, or by coagulating them
- Even by chelating trace elements indispensable to the cellular functioning (as the calcium or the magnesium)

The immediate or secondary necrosis (by more progressive diffusion into depth or by concomitant toxic effect) explain the macroscopic lesions of the tissues of the various eye structures (eyelids, conjunctiva, cornea, even iris or the ocular lens) that are specific to the chemical burn.

3.4 The Mechanisms of the Chemical Burn During the Contact Between the Aggressor and the Eye

Fig. 3.52 Phospholipids and cellular membrane structure

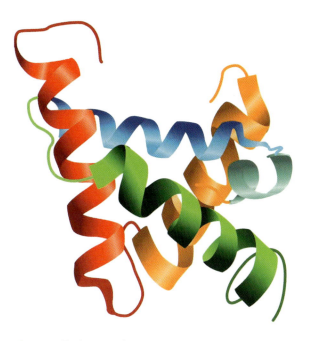

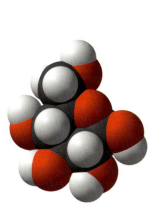

Fig. 3.53 Glucose

Fig. 3.54 Tertiary protein structure

Finally, we could sum up the action of corrosives on biological material to three levels of interaction:

- Modification of the balances of chemical reactivity: acid–base or redox reactions
- Modification of biological molecules (by reactions of addition or substitution), for instance, by alkylating agents or as a consequence of a coagulation of proteins
- Disappearing of an active entity for cases such as chelating agents (for instance, the fluor ion) or solvents

3.4 The Mechanisms of the Chemical Burn During the Contact Between the Aggressor and the Eye

3.4.1 The Different Elementary Types of Chemical Reactivity

The analysis of the various characteristic reagent functions of the irritant or corrosive molecules and the nature of the biological constituents leads to the identification of a restricted number of reagent couples as mentioned in Sect. 3.2.2. In practice, there are six types of elementary reactions:

- Acid–base reaction
- Redox reaction
- Addition
- Substitution
- Chelating reaction
- Solvation

The acid–base couple is the most known because of the massive and ubiquitous use of the acids and bases in work environment as well as in homelife during chemical assaults. But it is not the only cause of ocular irritations or corrosions. An oxidizer or a reducing agent can also generate lesions to tissues.

What happens between both protagonists in this case? The oxidizer is going "to seek" from the reducer the transfer with definitive title of one or several electrons to complete its orbitals and so acquire a more stable external electronic cover. An oxidizer can answer a reducer and conversely (Fig. 3.55).

This sketch enables the understanding of the notion of exchange between the chemical aggressor and the target biological constituents of the eye. According to the type of reactive function of the aggressor and thus the type of elementary reaction with the target molecules, different types of entities will be exchanged. This may involve electrons for a redox reaction, ions for an acid–base reaction or for a chelating reaction, atoms or molecules for additions or substitutions.

This notion of exchange appeals to the concept of acceptor and donor. The chemical aggressor and the target can alternately be either the donor or the acceptor.

As mentioned above, an acid or a base that does not express in the same way is thus totally disarmed with regard to an oxidizer or a reducer. Any chemical reactivity between them is thus totally impossible.

Nevertheless, some molecular structures may have several various elementary functions (Fig. 3.56).

For instance, hydrogen peroxide H_2O_2 is both acid and oxidizing.

Hydrofluoric acid is a particular illustration because it associates the elementary mechanism of the acid and the mechanism of a chelation causing a major toxic effect.

Chelation can be defined as the appropriation of mainly metallic atoms by a molecular entity, the size of which is often bigger. It is another example of

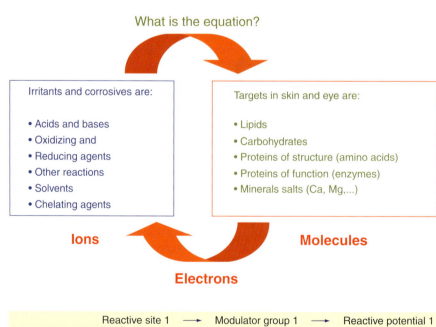

Fig. 3.55 Mechanism of chemical burn

Fig. 3.56 Reactive potential of a chemical substance

elementary chemical reactivity that may hurt the biological structures in contact.

HF is a partial dissociated acid (pK = 3.2). It releases 1,000 times less H⁺ ions in water than the same quantity of hydrochloric acid (pK = –2.2).

Therefore, the measurement of the pH alone is not enough to inform about the aggressiveness of this acid.

Nevertheless, the lesions provoked by HF are dreadful and may even endanger the vital prognosis of the individual because of the cardiac complications that it can engender in case of associated facial projection. Why? Simply because to the initial destruction of the structures of the eye by its acid potential (ion H⁺), is added the chelating and toxic action of the fluoride ion (F⁻) (Fig. 3.57). This action will develop gradually, in situ in the layers of the cornea, as the HF breaks up. This results in a deep damage with a necrotic character.

In this particular case, one F⁻ ion chelates two Ca⁺⁺ or Mg⁺⁺ ions so disrupting the biochemical metabolisms until the occurrence of cellular death and the necrosis of tissues. It is a movement of physiological balance. This mechanism explains the first historic reflex to strengthen the contributions in ions Ca⁺⁺ or Mg⁺⁺ ions to answer the need of chelation of the fluoride ion. This resulted, in the last past years, in the generalization of therapy protocols mainly using calcium gluconate.

All in all, the conditions of the reactivity of a chemical "aggressor" are bound to the intimate features of its constituting atoms. Molecules, whether they are irritants or corrosives, fill in not only specific conditions of "interlocutor" but also of sufficient energy level as we mentioned in Fig. 3.58.

Such a more mechanistic approach of the reactional context is called "reflexive toxicology" [2] because it requires second thought and reasoning. It is not only indispensable any more to learn "by heart" lists of effects without understanding why or how they work. It is a very effective solution, which enables an important economy of means and time.

3.4.2 Energy Dimension of Chemical Burns

For a long time, chemists have had an extremely accurate knowledge not only of the type but also the energy intensity of chemical reactions.

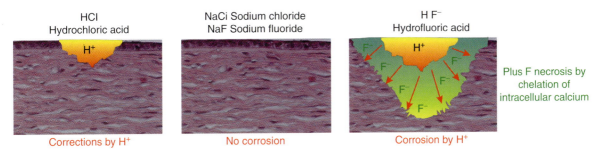

Fig. 3.57 HF burn mechanism

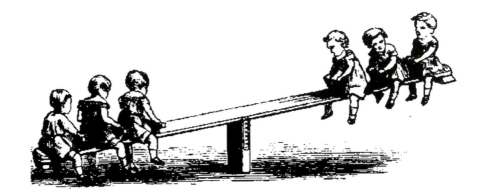

Fig. 3.58 Energy level

A chemical burn can be conceived only between two chemical entities in interaction with each other, one acting as the "donor" the other one as the "acceptor." It is the strength of the corrosive aggressor that affects the weakness of its biochemical target, until it consumes it completely. Then, the aggressor attacks the species of hardly superior energy level and so on until exhaustion of its own concentration (Fig. 3.58).

For example, a strong acid can only act on a weak base. If the base was stronger than the acid, the base would react by consuming the acid. An acid of given energy level (pK) is going to consume all the bases of weaker energy level (pK of a bigger value) beginning with the most remote level. Lobes represent the concentration involved by the aggressor on one hand and by the potential biochemical targets on the other hand (Fig. 3.59).

For a corrosive attack of the cornea, the biological targets will be among others the residues of the amino acids of the tissues proteins.

In summary, in order to understand the mechanism of chemical burns, it is necessary to be able to integrate all the previously detailed data, the interaction of which is summed up in the following plan (Fig. 3.60).

The general structure of a molecule is, most of the time, carbon. It can be considered as a main structure

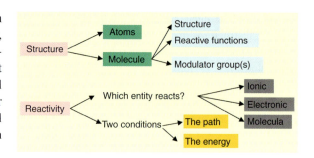

Fig. 3.60 Structure and function relationship

on which are "connected" one or several functional groups. These groups are responsible for the type of chemical reactivity of the substance: acid, basic, oxidizing, reducing.

The level of expression of the intensity of this reactivity can be increased or decreased by one or several atoms or groups of atoms called "modulators."

3.4.3 Key Parameters of Chemical Burns

Some of these fundamental notions will be also summed up in Chap. 6 under the more applied perspective of the pathophysiological mechanisms of chemical eye burns.

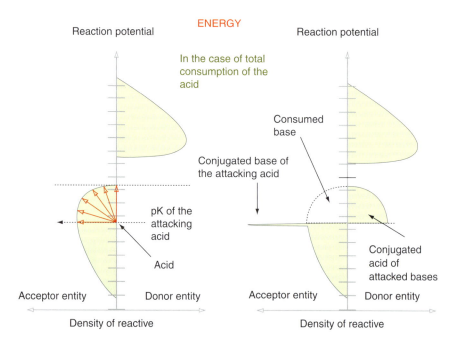

Fig. 3.59 Donor–acceptor relationship

3.4 The Mechanisms of the Chemical Burn During the Contact Between the Aggressor and the Eye

3.4.3.1 Danger Resulting of the Nature of the Involved Chemical

Solid Form

During an eye projection of a solid chemical, there is a double effect:

- Physical aggression, which is translated by an erosion of the surface of the cornea
- Chemical aggression, which is translated by a cellular necrosis

The following experiment illustrates this problem. It shows the time that is necessary for the dissolution of a soda pellet in water during the simulation of a simple wash (with a 150 mL/min debit). These observations show that it takes 2 min and 30 s so that the soda pellet dissolves completely during a continuous wash with the excitement of a stirring magnet. Without stirring, it takes 3 min and 30 s. Knowing that some solid particles dissolve more or less quickly, it will then be necessary to prolong the wash and to examine attentively the conjunctival sacs and the surface of the cornea with a slitlamp to make sure that any particle was well eliminated.

The pH curve shows a weak evolution. It's the same with the temperature curve (Fig. 3.61).

Viscosity

The viscosity is responsible for a covering effect, which makes the simple passive wash more difficult, because the product sticks on the contact area (Figs. 3.62 and 3.63).

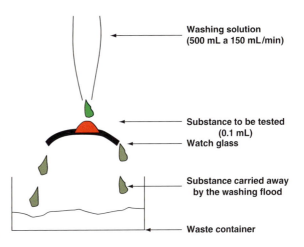

Fig. 3.62 Viscosity measurement schema

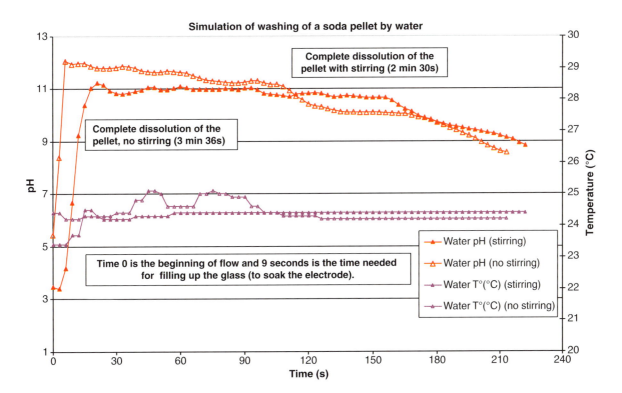

Fig. 3.61 Soda pellet simulation of water washing

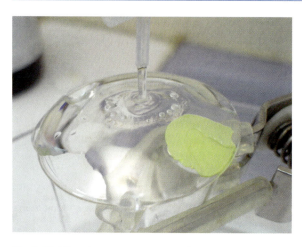

Fig. 3.63 Viscosity measurement experimental setup

Exothermic Reaction

Certain products, in contact with water, react and release corrosive products. This reaction develops more or less violently according to the involved chemical agent. This rise of temperature may aggravate the burn. Some examples:

- The powerful reducing agents such as sodium and lithium
- The anhydrous form of the acids such as the icy acetic acid or the sulfuric acid when concentrated beyond 96%
- Alkylaluminums

$$TiCl_4 + 4H_2O \longrightarrow Ti(OH)_4 + 4HCl$$

Fig. 3.64 Titanium tetrachloride

- Titanium salts ($TiCl_4$) (Fig. 3.64)
- Chlorosilanes (trichloromethylsilane)
- Bore (BF_3)

Titanium Tetrachloride

When in contact with water or any other aqueous solution, $TiCl_4$ releases some hydrochloric acid (Fig. 3.64).

An in vitro manipulation helps to objectify the variations of pH and of temperature when we add to 1 mL of tetrachloride of titanium, an increasing volume of water then, in comparison, an increasing volume of Diphoterine®.

The reaction instantaneously generates a release of energy and an increase of temperature. Very quickly, when adding 5 mL of water or Diphoterine®, this exothermic effect decreases, because of dilution, and the temperature returns to 20 °C.

On this purely physical aspect water and Diphoterine® have the same effect. However, there is a big difference on the chemical side. From this point of view, Diphoterine®, with a very low volume added, restores the pH toward the acceptable physiologic zone very quickly, while water maintains a very corrosive pH (Fig. 3.65).

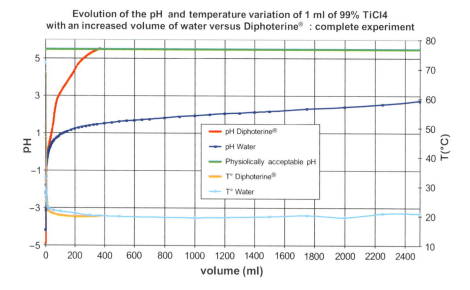

Fig. 3.65 Titanium tetrachloride experimental washing

3.4 The Mechanisms of the Chemical Burn During the Contact Between the Aggressor and the Eye

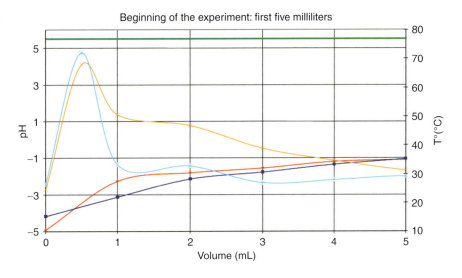

Fig. 3.66 Titanium tetrachloride experimental washing (zoom on first 5 mL)

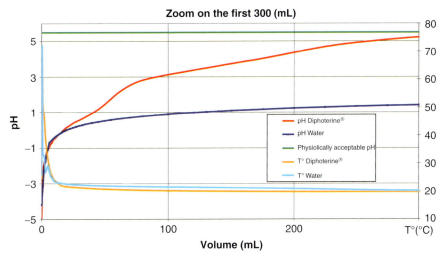

Fig. 3.67 Titanium tetrachloride experimental washing (zoom on first 300 mL)

Moreover, the speed of washing is a factor that is not as decisive for thermal burns as it is for chemical burns.

For the latter, on the other hand, the fundamental element of aggressiveness is the persistence of pH values out of the physiological zone.

Let us look closer at the very beginning of the manipulation, for more precision on the look of curves by zoom effect on the first 5 mL (Fig. 3.66).

In the same way, let us look at the first 300 mL (Fig. 3.67).

Trichloromethylsilane

Like titanium tetrachloride, when in contact with water or any other aqueous solution, trichloromethylsilane releases some hydrochloric acid (Fig. 3.68).

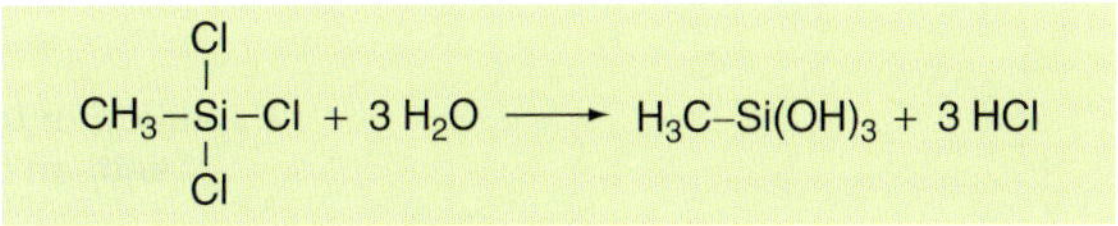

$$CH_3-\underset{\underset{Cl}{|}}{\overset{\overset{Cl}{|}}{Si}}-Cl + 3\,H_2O \longrightarrow H_3C-Si(OH)_3 + 3\,HCl$$

Fig. 3.68 Trichloromethylsilane

The same release of energy occurs with trichloromethylsilane than with titanium tetrachloride. We observed the same conclusions than in the previous paragraph using water compared Diphoterine® (Fig. 3.69).

Boron Trifluoride

In contact with water, BF_3 forms some boron hydroxide $(B(OH)_3)$ and releases some hydrofluoric acid (Fig. 3.70).

Fig. 3.69 Trichloromethylsilane experimental washing

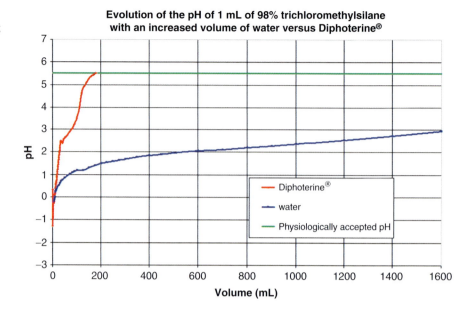

Fig. 3.70 Boron trifluoride

$$BF_3 + 3H_2O \longrightarrow B(OH)_3 + 3HF$$

In the following experiment of dosage, we can observe that water has only an effect of passive dilution with a pH and a pF, which remain low in spite of the increasing addition of a big quantity of water (Fig. 3.71).

On the contrary, the increasing addition of Hexafluorine® very quickly restores both the pH and the pF toward the physiologically acceptable level.

Other types of chemicals, as concentrated corrosives and particularly the acids, may react with water by a release of heat.

The heating produced during the contact of a concentrated corrosive and water can be experimentally observed in a beaker. The effect can be observed in statics or in dynamics during a simulation of wash.

Sulfuric Acid

With the example of very concentrated sulfuric acid (H_2SO_4) in contact with water, the solvation releases a very big heating of more than 90°C (Fig. 3.72).

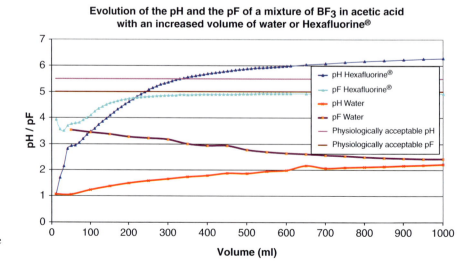

Fig. 3.71 Boron trifluoride experimental washing

3.4 The Mechanisms of the Chemical Burn During the Contact Between the Aggressor and the Eye

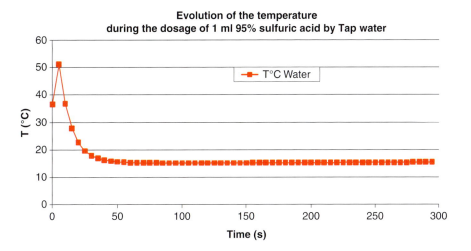

Fig. 3.72 Sulfuric acid experimental washing

If during a static dilution, the temperature is very high, it is no more the same there during a dynamic wash.

In dynamics (Fig. 3.73), the external wash enables the measurement of the effect of mechanical draining of the wash associated with the effect diminution of the temperature, which is exponential, and thus very fast (Fig. 3.74).

We then observe that, thanks to the wash, temperature reaches no more than 50 degrees over a few seconds. Usually considered as "icy," this very concentrated, even totally anhydride, acid reacts with water via the formation of hydrogen bonds, which cause an exothermic reaction, a sign of a molecular excitement and a variation of entropy (Fig. 3.74).

This heating is not as big with soda (Fig. 3.75):

When in contact with some skin or an eye, the very concentrated corrosives, dissolve the water of tissues. Before they really lead to a chemical burn, or simultaneously, these very concentrated corrosives can cause a burn by dehydration and/or by thermal effect.

Once more, this justifies the necessity of beginning the wash as soon as possible.

3.4.3.2 Risk Factors in Relation with the Conditions of Use

Concentration of the Chemical

The chemical burn is the expression of a chemical ability to react between two molecules, a xenobiotic one and a biochemical tissues one. An acid can only affect the eye if it finds some chemical structures of basic nature in the cornea. It's the same for the attack of an oxidizing agent toward reducing cellular molecules. Generally speaking, in a chemical reaction, there is always a donor entity and an acceptor entity. For more details see Sect. 3.4.2.

As the reactions develop one by one, the consumption is made from molecules to molecules. The local reaction continues until exhaustion of the molecules in presence,

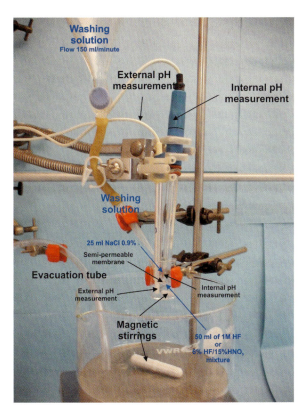

Fig. 3.73 Dynamic wash experimental setup

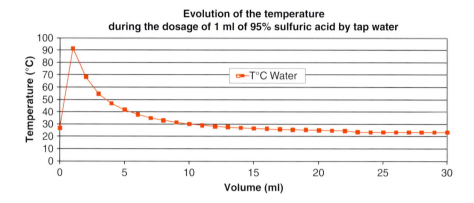

Fig. 3.74 Sulfuric acid external dynamic rinsing simulation

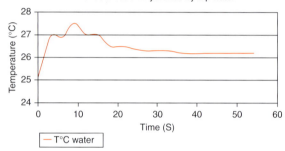

Fig. 3.75 Sodium hydroxide external rinsing simulation

on one side or the other one. In the case of the corrosive aggression, until exhaustion of the xenobiotic aggressor the power of which, on the reactivity scale, is always, by definition, superior to that of its tissue target. The levels of cellular structures will so successively be destroyed, from the surface toward the depth. The macroscopic lesions will be more and more spread and deep.

Depending on the relative levels of energy and the concentration of the aggressor, the burn will or will not develop, until dramatic situations for very powerful and very concentrated corrosives.

Unlike that case, if the concentration of the aggressor is weak, few or no tissue molecules will be consumed. The anatomical damages will be superficial and easily repairable, or even nonexistent.

This sets up the concept of concentration threshold from which we are going to be able to observe the expression of the reaction between the chemical aggressor and its target molecule and thus the appearance of the burn. For the eye and in the case of acids and bases, this concentration threshold is around 0.2N as mentioned in Sect. 3.2.4.2 (Fig. 3.46). It is then more easily understood that a diluted corrosive will develop an only irritant potential because there are not enough reactive entities.

Beyond a certain concentration threshold, the difference of aggressiveness will be directly proportional to the intrinsic energy intensity of the chemical agent quantified on the various scales described in Sect. 3.2.4.

On the opposite side, the small attacks repeated by a very concentrated irritant can accumulate microlesions that could be quite severe in the end. For instance, the more we concentrate a weak acid such as acetic acid, the more aggressive we make it. The icy acetic acid is a strong corrosive because it is moreover totally anhydride. When in contact with cellular biological liquids, it literally pumps all the water and provokes a necrosis of tissues.

Globally, this approach asks another question: what is the limit of the reversibility of the burn. This limit would be the resultant of several factors:

- The nature of the chemical agent
- Its concentration
- The time of contact

Phenomenon of the Diffusion of Corrosives in Relation with Their Concentration

The diffusion of a xenobiotic agent depends both on its chemical and physical properties:

- Physically, it is easy to conceive that a sticky and solid product or with a big molar mass penetrates much less further inside the tissues than a light and fluid, more or less hydrophilic or lipophilic substance.

3.4 The Mechanisms of the Chemical Burn During the Contact Between the Aggressor and the Eye

- Chemically, according to the nature of reactivity, the penetration will be more or less easy and/or will delay. This results in either immediate or massive lesions as it happens with strong acids or more delayed and evolutionary burns as it happens with soda or hydrofluoric acid.

Here follows the simulation of the ocular penetration of various corrosives according to their concentration. The experiment consists in depositing the chemical on a semipermeable membrane (Figs. 3.76 and 3.77) in contact with a 420 mosmol/kg salt solution, in order to mimic corneal osmolarity and in the observation of the penetration of the corrosive into the salt solution in relation with time (Fig. 3.78).

At 0.2M, soda penetrates very little and the final pH does not exceed 10. This corresponds to the data of the table of prediction of the irritant or corrosive power (see Sect. 3.2.4.2 and Fig. 3.46).

At 0.2M, sulfuric acid already penetrates with a resulting pH of 2.5 (Fig. 3.79). It is a diacid. It can thus release twice more aggressive entities. Even in weak concentration, it quickly generates lesions.

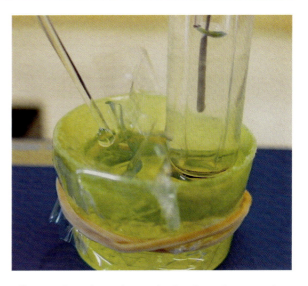

Fig. 3.76 Experimental set to simulate the ocular penetration

Time of Contact

The time of contact of the corrosive with the surface of the eye is also a key factor of the gravity of a chemical burn.

When two reagent chemical substances are put together in a test tube, the chemical reaction is almost

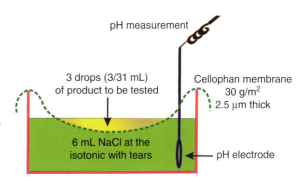

Fig. 3.77 Schema of ocular penetration experimental set

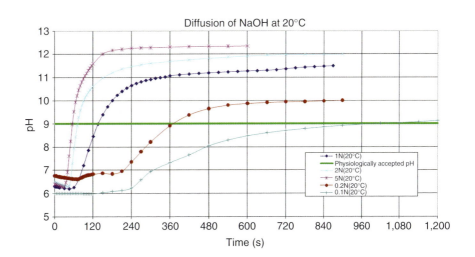

Fig. 3.78 Diffusion of sodium hydroxide

Fig. 3.79 Diffusion of sulfuric acid

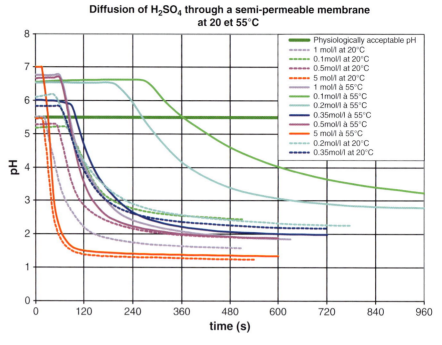

immediate. The situation is a little bit different when a corrosive gets in touch with a biological tissue.

The epithelium, the most superficial cellular layer of the cornea of the eye, is chemically less resistant than the keratinized epidermis of the skin. However, during ocular accidents, we know that it takes a few seconds for the first lesions to appear. This delay is bound to multiple factors, winking reflex, protective and diluting effect of the lachrymal liquid, effect of sweeping of the palpebral movements. After a short period, a kinetic of diffusion will set up in a variable way according to the nature of the corrosive.

All in all, in an optimal way, an effective capture and a definitive neutralization of the corrosive within the 10 s following the contact with the eye can guarantee the absence of lesions and so avoid the burn. By intervening within the first minute, the eye chemical burn shall be avoided or minimized. Beyond this first minute, the lesions gradually and inexorably settle down. This does not mean that there is no more profit to intervene! It is what demonstrates the study of a clinical case of burn with late care [3, 4].

Finally, Chaps. 5 and 6 will develop the experimental results of the penetration of various corrosive compounds through the cornea, up to the anterior chamber, in the contact of the lens (see Sect. 5.1.6).

Temperature

Temperature facilitates:

- The ability of chemicals to react
- The speed of penetration into tissues
- Reaction with the cells

It creates a dynamic effect, by increasing the average speed of excitement of the reagent (chemical substances/constituents of the skin and the eye) and thus by increasing the number of efficient shocks between molecules. In the same way, as previously studied, another aggravating factor such as the concentration of the chemical aggressor increases the number of effective shocks. Another phenomenon to consider is the vasodilatation bound to the heat; it is the resulting edema of the tissues. In the experiment (Fig. 3.80), the diffusion of 55°C preheated soda is faster than the diffusion of 20°C soda. This effect is particularly important for a 1N concentration, knowing that at 5N the difference is less marked because the effect of mass naturally makes the diffusion faster.

With a less important concentration but a higher temperature, a chemical can turn out corrosive. Thus, it can have similar effects to those obtained with a more important concentration but with an ambient temperature (20°C).

3.5 Practical Conclusions in Order to Manage the Optimal Chemical Decontamination of an Eye

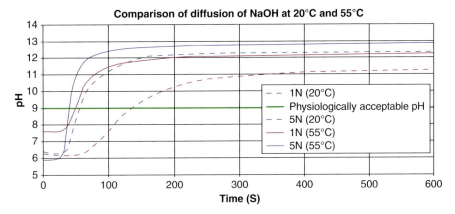

Fig. 3.80 Comparative diffusion of sodium hydroxide

On the other hand, proportionally, the influence of temperature is less important for an already very concentrated substance.

Pressure

The pressure can sharply facilitate the penetration of the corrosive into the depth of the eye. By a physical phenomenon, the pressure entails a mechanical disintegration of the tissues. This will aggravate all the lesions.

3.5 Practical Conclusions in Order to Manage the Optimal Chemical Decontamination of an Eye

The gravity of an ocular chemical burn is due to multiple factors.

It is, of course, in touch relative to the intrinsic chemical nature of the substance but it also depends on the physical conditions of use.

These practical notions can have consequences at several levels:

- Primary prevention in the workplace or in domestic environment
- Precocity, relevance, and efficiency of the various parameters of the indispensable and specific decontamination to set up within the seconds following an eye projection

By optimizing each of these parameters, the initial burn can be avoided or its importance be minimized.

Considering the fundamental notions developed above, what conclusions can be stated using these theoretical and experimental data in order to define an optimal process for the decontamination of an ocular chemical projection?

What are the technical means indispensable for the emergency care of an ocular chemical burn? How to be rational and efficient just after contact?

3.5.1 The First Reflex: The Passive Wash Including Dilution and Mechanical Draining

The first reflex is dilution and mechanical draining with water. It is still efficient for the least aggressive chemicals and the least concentrated substances.

What happens when considering the mechanistics developed in the previous paragraphs?

A simple in vitro experiment enables the observation of the effect of dilution by water of concentrated corrosives such as soda or sulfuric acid (Fig. 3.81):

In spite of adding a big quantity of water, pH remains around 2, which is very corrosive.

During the contact between the chemical aggressor and the biological molecules constituting the cellular structures of an eye, the reactivity develops from molecules to molecules, until complete consumption of all the corrosive molecules. Thus, the less concentrated the corrosive, the smaller the number of biological molecules consumed and the smaller the cellular destruction. Similarly, during the passive dilution of a water wash, less and less entities are available to cause lesions. Nevertheless, even in a diluted solution,

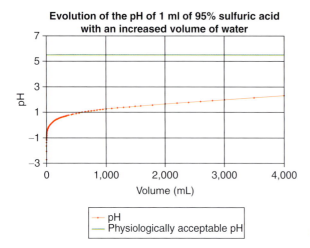

Fig. 3.81 Evolution of the pH of sulfuric acid

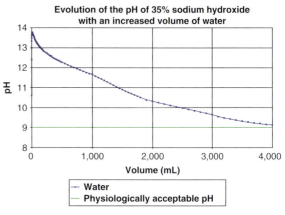

Fig. 3.82 pH evolution of sodium hydroxide

a corrosive molecule keeps all of its own reacting potential.

Thus the lesions to tissues become less and less noticeable but they will still develop. This is the main argument supporting the need of a prolonged 15–20 min wash.

3.5.2 Consequences of a Passive Washing: A Longer Time of Action

The reasoning developed in the previous paragraphs justifies the old international consensus on the recommendation of a 15–20 min prolonged wash when using water.

But why is it essential to continue the wash after 5 or 10 min? Because there is still a high destructive potential and lesions are still developing. This evidence shows the insufficiency of a simple effect of mechanical draining and passive dilution of a water wash.

Figure 3.82 illustrates this with a logarithmic curve ending with an asymptote.

Knowing well such dilution techniques, the scientist in chemistry will search for a better solution than such a slow, gradual, and partial phenomenon.

Of course the effect of mechanical draining from the tissue's surface gradually eliminates about 90% of the corrosive. But the remaining 10% are still aggressive enough to cause the evident severeness of some chemical burns, which had first been early and widely washed with water anyway [5]. Moreover, it is well known that about 250 mL remain on the surface of a naked body after complete immersion. For an eye, the winking reflex drives almost all the substance out except for a volume of about one drop that reaches the cornea. Therefore, it is easy to understand that chemical burns are due to very small quantities of chemicals.

3.5.3 The Concept of Active Wash

While keeping the principle of washing as a dilution, the chemist would search for a solution to get an immediate and complete neutralization. This is the actual goal of searching for solutions of active wash.

However, about 200 years ago, Thénard and Gay-Lussac were the pioneers who decided to concentrate an HF solution and to study the very specific characteristics of both its physical and its chemical properties. They have noticed that the use of a solution of diluted potash could stop both pains and burns caused by HF. Why was this brand-new concept abandoned so quickly? Is the exothermic characteristic of the reaction the only cause of this abandon and is it only a myth? The limit of effectiveness of passive washing is probably the principal explanation.

Since a very long time, the chemists are using solutions of weak acids or weak bases to neutralize, respectively, strong bases and strong acids. They equipped their laboratories with bottles of weak acids and weak bases to neutralize ocular or skin projections.

Despite good intentions, the results have not always been remarkable! At first, it would have been necessary to know the nature of the chemical, then to know exactly the strength of the reaction, while also considering the exothermic character of the reaction, the lack

Fig. 3.83 pH evolution of different corrosives with addition of Diphoterine®

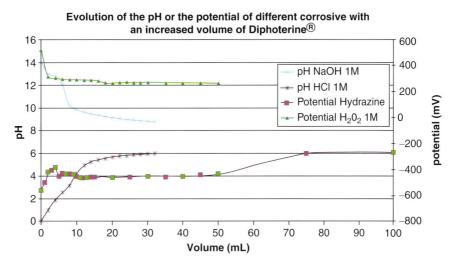

of sterility of the solution, and, more especially, the risk of errors.

For these reasons one thinks of using buffer solutions. What is a buffer solution?

A buffer solution is a solution which resists change of pH upon addition of small amounts of acid or base, or upon dilution. It is made with material pairs:

- Weak acid and a soluble salt containing the conjugate base of the weak acid
- Weak base and a soluble salt containing the conjugate acid of the weak base

For example, the resistive action is the result of the equilibrium between the weak acid (HA) and its conjugate base (A⁻):

$$HA(aq) + H_2O \leftrightarrow H_3O^+(aq) + A^-(aq)$$

The best effectiveness of a buffer is reached when the pH of the solution is close to the pK$_a$ of the weak acid and conversely for the weak base.

If one washes, by error, a strong acid projection with a weak acid like, for example, the boric acid, the benefit will be null. The strong acid will not be washed at all.

All these problems can be solved in a modern way by the conception and the realization of amphoteric solutions available in sterile containers. (Amphoteric solutions can react with antagonistic couples of corrosives such as acid/base, oxidizing/reducing agents). These methods, moreover a chemical washing and dilution at the surface of the cornea, propose a dynamic additive effect via chemical reactivity of the offending chemical.

The idea is to bind the aggressive chemical agent quicker than it could react with the biological component of the cornea, preventing and induced damage.

Beyond the simple polyvalent dilution of a water wash, the wash (Fig. 3.83) of various types of corrosives by Diphoterine® an amphoteric agent shows the need and profit of the use of an active answer.

The experimental simulation of a chemical burn (Figs. 3.84 and 3.85) is stated on a corrosive such as some 1M soda in contact for 3 min with the semipermeable membrane representing the cornea. It favorably shows the time gained, thanks to a solution that physically and chemically helps the pH of the aqueous humor to get back to the safe zone. Here, the point is not only to show the mechanical draining effect at the surface of the membrane/cornea (which quickly restores the pH to a normal value), but also to show how the internal decontamination of a corrosive is important and difficult. The internal decontamination will deal with the amount of corrosive that might have already penetrated into the anterior chamber of the eye.

It is noticeable that an increase of the osmotic pressure of the wash solution that is used can lower the time required to restore the pH to a physiologically acceptable zone. Therefore, it shortens the required washing time (the gap is due to osmolarity) (Fig. 3.86):

The use of a solution that is able to react with the corrosive will, in an even more remarkable way, reduce the time needed to restore the pH to a safe zone (the gap is

3.6 What is Now the Extent of Our Knowledge About Ocular Chemical Burns?

We are now able to know the intimate nature of the chemical aggression by an irritant or a corrosive on the "fragile" biological structures of an eye. We can also evaluate the strength of this aggression.

We better understand the kinetics of spreading and the histological processes of destruction of the different ocular tissues. The pathophysiology of chemical lesions, in case of an ocular burn, will be strongly illustrated, thanks to new technologies which can bring the experimental evidence of the theories developed in the following chapters.

We all know that the time available before the settlement of burns is very short and very valuable. Particularly in professional environment, we must be ready to react not only in case of an acid or a base projection but also when chemical reagents, such as oxidizing, reducing, or chelating agents, and so on, might be involved, because these other aggressors are widely used in industry and might cause severe chemical ocular accidents. So short delay for decontamination and polyvalence are key parameters of the expected efficiency of the chemical decontamination. These notions are gathered and illustrated in Fig. 3.87.

The universal and unconditional use of water is due to its polyvalence, its effect of mechanical draining and dilution at the surface of the tissues. However, water has limits. It requires an extremely fast intervention with the necessity of using a huge quantity to get results that might be neither reproduced nor reproducible. Therefore, the use of water does not guarantee a safe situation, especially when corrosives are concentrated.

When using specific chemical concepts, we are now able to conceive effective practical answers so that really efficient first aid wash solutions can be available for victims of eye projections, in case of an emergency.

The approach developed in this chapter already shows some axis of prevention and optimal care of the ocular chemical accident:

- Precocity of the intervention.
- Effect of dilution and mechanical draining.
- Polyvalence because of the diversity of substances and often because of the misknowledge of the precise composition of the irritant or corrosive chemicals involved.

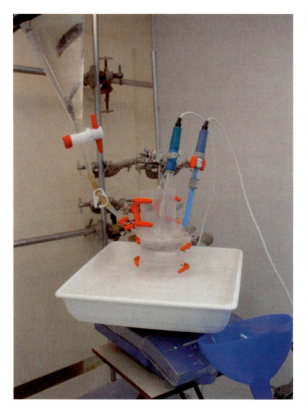

Fig. 3.84 Experimental setup for simulation of a chemical burn

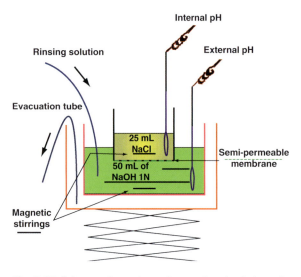

Fig. 3.85 Schema of experimental setup for simulation of a chemical burn

due to amphoteric property). Experimentally, it is noticeable that the hypertonicity reduces this time by a 30% factor only; while an active and safe neutralization – with the meaning of the amphoteric solution used in this experiment – reduces the washing time by a factor 4.

3.6 What is Now the Extent of Our Knowledge About Ocular Chemical Burns?

Fig. 3.86 Evolution of ocular pH with different decontamination solutions

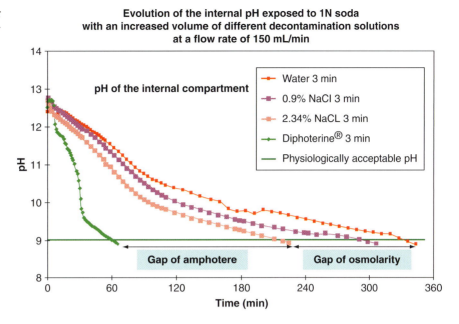

Fig. 3.87 Summary of chemical burn knowledge

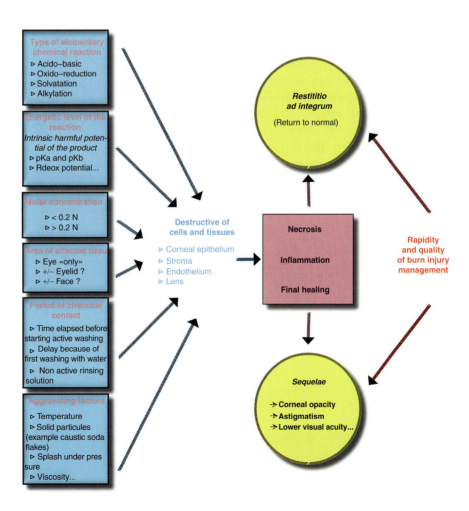

- Innocuousness: the solution must not be irritant or toxic, have no deleterious effect, must cause no sensitization, and be sterile and compatible with secondary ophthalmologic treatments.

In the following chapters, we will study the experimental and clinical dimensions due to the gathering of a modern knowledge mixing chemistry and medicine.

Beyond the basic requirements mentioned above, the difference in efficiency of a wash solution is bound to a real ability to react and thus to control the aggressiveness of all the irritants and corrosives on the side of their specific elementary reactivity:

- Acid–base reaction
- Redox
- Chelation
- Addition
- Substitution
- Solvation

In practice, this ability to control the aggressor supplies some precious extra seconds in order to start an efficient decontamination. Without requiring huge quantities of wash liquid because the efficiency can be reached even with a small amount of the solution to use and without needing one duration of washing as prolonged as that of water.

The last consequence is that the chemical lesion is avoided or minimized. This facilitates the simplicity of the follow-up care in case of a secondary medical treatment. All these elements bring the patients real advantages:

- Very early analgesic effect that makes a careful wash more comfortable and efficient and avoids blepharospasm
- Quickness and simplicity of evolution
- Diminution of the risk not only of functional sequelae but also of psychological damages

References

1. Liao, C.-C., Rossignol, A.M.: Burns **26**, 422 (2000)
2. Burgher, F., Mathieu, L., Blomet, J.: Le Risque chimique et la Santé au Travail [Chemical risk and occupational medicine]. Prevor editions 1996
3. Merle, H., Donnio, A., Ayeboua, L., Michel, F., Thomas, F., Ketterle, J., Leonard, C., Josset, P., Gerard, M.: Alkali ocular burns in Martinique (French West Indies) Evaluation of the use of an amphoteric solution as the rinsing product. Burns **31**(2), 205–211 (2005)
4. Gérard, M., Merle, H., Chiambaretta, F., Rigal, D., Schrage, N.: An amphoteric rince used in the emergency treatment of a serious ocular burn. Burns **7**, 670–673 (2002)
5. Hall, A.H., HI, Maibach: Water decontamination of chemical skin/eye splashes: a critical review. Cutan Ocul Toxicol **25**(2), 67–83 (2006)
6. Burgher, F., Blomet, J., Mathieu, M.: La magie des solvants, Principes, Toxicologie, Risque Ecologique, Solutions alternatives [Magics Solvents, Principals, Toxicology, Ecological risk, Alternative Solutions]. Prevor editions 1998

Histology and Physiology of the Cornea

Max Gérard and Patrice Josset

4.1 Corneal Functions

The cornea enables the penetration of rays of light inside the eye, thanks to completely particular optical capacities allied to its great fragility largely due to its distant origin within the aquatic species. We will see how the histology of the cornea helps to understand this permanent miracle.

Doted of a refractive capacity of about 43 dioptres, the cornea is a sphere-cylinder like lens and counts for two thirds of the refractive power of an eye at resting state.

4.2 Anatomy Reminder

With a size of about 1.3 cm^2 and an average diameter of 11.5 mm in adulthood, the cornea has an ovoid shape with a horizontal axis on its front side and is circular on its back side. It is 0.5-mm thick at the center and 1-mm thick on the edge. As shown by modern measurements, the shape of the cornea can differ for different individuals. On its edge there is the limbus that partly has the same characteristics and ensures the junction with the totally opaque sclera, which surrounds the entire eyeball.

M. Gérard (✉)
Medical director of Head and Neck Unit, Ophtalmologist,
Cayenne Hospital, Cayenne, French Guiana
e-mail: gerardmax@caramail.com

P. Josset
In charge of courses on the history of the medicine,
Curator of the Dupuytren museum Paris, Anatomopathologist,
"Armand Trousseau" Children's Hospital, Paris, France
e-mail: patrice.josset@trs.ap-hop-paris.fr

4.3 Histology

The cornea is made up of five layers [1]:

1. The epithelium and its basement membrane
2. Bowman's membrane
3. The corneal stroma
4. Descemet's membrane
5. The endothelial cells

4.3.1 The Epithelium and Its Basement Membrane

The corneal epithelium is made of stratified and keratinless scale-like and junction-like cells. These cells are arranged on 4–6 layers at the central part and 4–8 layers on the edge of the cornea. Their combined thickness is about 50–60 μm representing about 10% of the whole thickness of the cornea. The structure and function of the epithelium strictly depends on the lacrymal secretion that covers it and plays a big part in the preservation of the cells and in their transparency.

We will now study, from edge to center, the lacrymal secretion and the layers of the corneal epithelium.

4.3.1.1 The Lacrymal Secretion

It cannot be dissociated from the epithelium because they share optic and metabolic functions. The lacrymal secretion is made up of three layers, from outside to inside:

- A 0.1-μm thick superficial lipidic layer with a main function of reducing the speed of evaporation of the lacrymal secretion. This lipidic film can only be

secreted by the conjunctival tarsal cells located on the palpebral edge.
- A middle 7-μm thick aqueous layer secreted by the lacrymal glands, with an average debit of 1.2 μL/min.
- A deep layer rich in mucus and the origin of which is to be found in the conjunctival calyciform cells. This mucus is in relation with the apical epithelial cells via the glycocalyx. This interface between the lacrymal secretion and the epithelium influences the quality of the corneal surface. Indeed, the stability of the lacrymal secretion and the epithelial absorption of its metabolites both depend on the mucin and the apical expansions of the epithelial cells [2].

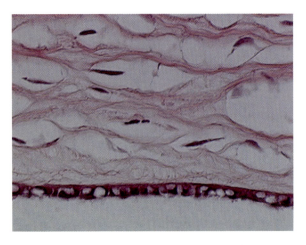

Fig. 4.2 Aspect of the cornea at the fourth month of pregnancy: the endothelial cells are dense and cubical

4.3.1.2 The Corneal Epithelium

It is formed very early in the ocular embryogenesis, at first as the simple epithelium, which is gradually replaced by the final form of epithelium: this latter is mostly made of malpighian epithelial cells but also contains non-epithelial lymphocytes (mostly T lymphocytes) and Langerhans cells (cells of presentation of the antigen), both playing a part in immunity. There are also melanocytes at the level of the basal layer. These non-epithelial cells can mainly be found at the level of the corneal edge, close to the limbus (Figs. 4.1 and 4.2).

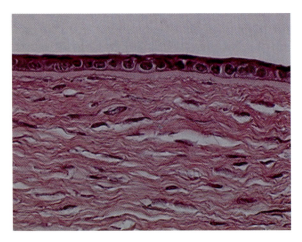

Fig. 4.1 Aspect of the cornea at the fourth month of pregnancy: the epithelium is constituted of one or two layers, the Bowman's membrane appears

4.3.1.3 The Superficial Cells

At the level of the superficial layer, itself made of two or three layers, the cells become more and more flattened and are 45-μm long and 4-μm thick. Their nucleus is stretched out along the long axis and is 25-μm long. Their cytoplasm contains three specific structures: contractile proteins, glycogen granules, and a very developed Golgi's apparatus.

Thanks to specular microscopy and electron scanning microscopy, some cells with various aspects have been identified: it could be different stages of differentiation and maturation of the superficial cells preceding their desquamation. Along their evolution, the metabolic activity of the superficial cells slows down until it stops. They are then evacuated into the lacrymal secretion.

The most superficial cells are the most mature ones, with a low metabolic activity, and they are going to desquamate. In electron scanning microscopy, the corneal surface looks like a mosaic of flattened and polygonal cells, with uneven sizes. Their nucleus is reduced to a few condensed chromatin clods.

Their cytoplasmic membrane is bristled up with microvillosities and micropilis. They increase the exchange surface with the lacrymal secretion and enable its fixing. Their lateral and basal cytoplasmic membranes have got junctional complexes uniting these superficial cells together. There are three types of junctional complexes:

- The desmosomes are very strong sticky junctions maintaining the mechanical cohesion of the

superficial cells. They are located along the lateral and basal membranes.
- The tight junctions are impermeable junctions maintaining the cellular cohesion and mostly represent a stopping system that prevents the passage of molecules and liquids from extracellular environment. They are located at the level of the apical part of the lateral cytoplasmic membranes.
- The gap junctions are communicating junctions, kinds of tunnels enabling the molecular exchanges between neighboring cells. They are spread in an anarchic way on the lateral and basal faces.

These junctional complexes all disappear during desquamation.

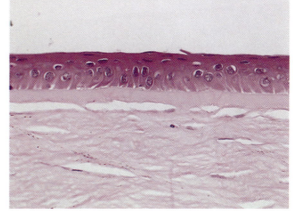

Fig. 4.4 Central part of corneal epithelium in adulthood 2

4.3.1.4 The Intermediate Cells

These are cells of transition between the basal and superficial cells. They constitute the thickest and biggest layer. They are polygonal cells, with a convex front side and a concave back side. They are arranged on two or three layers at the center and five to six layers on the edge. Their nucleus is active and stretched out along the big axis of the cell. Their cytoplasm contains a very developed Golgi's apparatus as well as tonofilaments (microtubules and keratin filaments) connected to the desmosomes. Their cytoplasmic membranes are only united desmosomes and gap junctions that enable both the unity of intermediate cells and the union of intermediate and basal cells (Figs. 4.3–4.5).

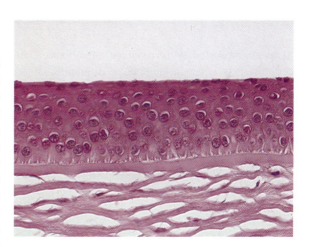

Fig. 4.5 Edge of corneal epithelium in adulthood

4.3.1.5 Basal Cells

Basal cells are the germinative cells of the corneal epithelium. They are 18-μm long cylindrical cells with a 10-μm diameter. They are arranged in one layer set on the basement membrane. Their nucleus is oval and oriented along the big axis of the cell (Fig. 4.6).

The stem cells of the basal cells are located at the level of the limbus, which come from centripetal migration. The daughter cells migrate to form the intermediate cells. Their cytoplasm, which is rich in glycogen and mitochondria, shows their high metabolic activity. It also contains a Golgi's apparatus, some microtubules, and some keratin filaments connected to each other by desmosomes and hemidesmosomes. Most of all this cytoplasm contains some actin

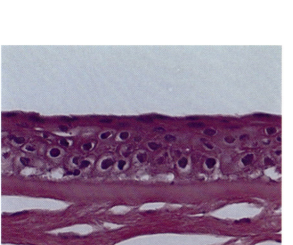

Fig. 4.3 Central part of corneal epithelium in adulthood 1

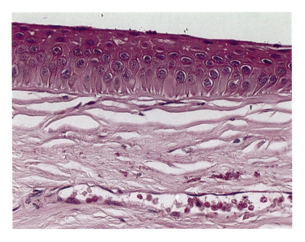

Fig. 4.6 Corneal back growth of epithelium after a burn: epithelial back growth, absence of the Bowman's membrane, and vascularization of the subjacent stroma

filaments supported by the basement membrane. They certainly play a part in the cellular migration. On its lateral and apical sides, their cytoplasmic membrane has desmosomes and gap junctions securing the cohesion of basal cells with each other and with the intermediate cells. Located on the basement membrane of the cell, the hemidesmosomes are part of the functional complex that enables the adhesion of epithelium to the subjacent structures.

4.3.1.6 The Basement Membrane

It separates the Bowman's membrane from the corneal epithelium. A 80-Å (angstrom) thick membrane, it is synthesized by the basal epithelial cells. It is bound to the basal cells and, in case of epithelial lesions of destruction; it guides and supports the back growth of the epithelium. It is constituted of type IV collagen and proteoglycans. The basement membrane has various functions: it guides the cellular migration, especially during the morphogenesis; it maintains the architecture of tissues, supporting the adhesion of cells; it sends and transmits information; it is a semipermeable membrane.

4.3.2 Bowman's Membrane

Bowman's membrane is an acellular membrane, which is 12-μm thick and located at the basement membrane and the stroma. During the fourth month of the embryonic period, the Bowman's membrane is certainly secreted by the epithelial cells, but it cannot be regenerated by these in case of a lesion. Therefore, a hurt to the Bowman's membrane results in a fibrous scar lesion. The Bowman's membrane is made of collagen fibers, mostly type I fibers randomly spread in a ground substance similar to the one of the corneal stroma.

4.3.3 The Stroma

It counts for about 90% of the global thickness of the human cornea. It is mainly made of an extracellular matrix rich in ground substance and of collagen lamellae the orientation of which is specific and complex. There are only a few cellular entities; some fibrocytes also named keratocytes, some lymphocytes, monocytes, some Langerhans cells as well as Schwann cells surrounding the very numerous axons that innerve the cornea. These cells account for less than 5% of the volume of the corneal stroma, which is not vascularized in normal conditions. Fibrocytes or keratocytes are flattened cells parallel to the collagen lamellae and to the cornea. They represent the resting state of the cell, which is similar to the one of the fibrocytes in other parts of the body. In case of a lesion, fibrocytes can migrate, while it is well known that they play a part in the secretion of the collagen fibers and of the ground substance (glycoproteins and proteoglycans).

There are about 200 2-μm thick collagen lamellae, piled up on each other in a very organized arrangement, which differs not only according to the corneal location but also according to the individual.

These lamellae play a part in both the transparency and the resistance to internal pressure of the eye.

4.3.3.1 Keratocytes

Keratocytes are cells of conjunctive type or fibrocytes. They account for 3–5% of the stromal volume. They are star-shaped cells, arranged in parallel to the corneal surface and to the collagen lamellae. Their nucleus is voluminous and flattened and has even edges. Their granular cytoplasm contains a few organelles, showing a weak metabolic or synthetic activity. Multiple cytoplasmic expansions spread from the nucleic region toward multiple directions and then reach some adjacent expansions of keratocytes via the tight junctions. Unlike ordinary fibrocytes, keratocytes can migrate during the scarring process. They gather on the edges of the lesion where they mute into fibroblast. Thus, they secure the synthesis of proteoglycans forming the extracellular matrix and of glycoproteins including collagen.

4.3.3.2 The Collagen Lamellae

There are about 200 to 250 collagen lamellae in the human corneal stroma. Each lamella is 2-μm thick and 9–260-μm wide. They are piled up on each other and have a very organized orientation. In the two thirds of the back of the stroma, the main axis of the collagen fibers of a lamella is perpendicular to the fibers of the lamellae that are above or below it. In the one third at the front of the stroma, the arrangement is less regular and the lamellae are set in an oblique arrangement to each other. Inside each lamella, the collagen fibrillae are parallel to each other, with even size and interspace. They are covered and thus separated from each other by some ground substance. Most of the stromal collagen (90%) is type I collagen, but a smaller part of it is types III and V. These lamellae play a double part:

- They secure and maintain the transparency of the cornea, mainly thanks to type V collagen, which influences the diameter of the collagen fibers and thus plays a part in the corneal transparency [3].
- They secure and maintain the mechanical resistance to the intraocular pressure, mainly thanks to type I and III collagen.

4.3.3.3 Ground Substance

The ground substance wraps the collagen lamellae and the cellular entities. It is constituted of glycoproteins and proteoglycans synthesized by the keratocytes. The main proteoglycans are made of glycosaminoglycans and are keratan sulfates – mostly type I – for 60% and chondroitin sulfates for 40%. These glycosaminoglycans are one of the factors of the corneal transparency, via the regulation of the stromal hydration. Thus, during endothelial disorders, the rise of the water content of the stroma causes an increase of the volume of the glycosaminoglycans. This makes the cornea thicker and breaks the even arrangement of the collage lamellae resulting in an alteration of the light transmission. At last, there is also some type VI collagen that might have a support function by separating the different constituents of the stroma.

4.3.3.4 Other Cells

The corneal stroma also contains Schwann cells, surrounding the corneal axons, and immunocompetent cells (T and B lymphocytes, monocytes, and Langerhans cells). These latter cells are very numerous at the level of the limbus close to small vessels, but there are also a few of them at the level of the one third at the front of the central corneal stroma [4].

4.3.4 Descemet's Membrane

It constitutes the basement membrane of the corneal endothelium, separating it from the stroma. It is a strong, amorphous, and elastic membrane. It is about 10 μm in adulthood. It is synthesized by the endothelial cells from the fourth month of embryonic life. The Descemet's membrane has got two distinct sides:

- A 3-μm thick front side corresponding to the striated embryonic portion secreted by the endothelial cells during gestation.
- A back granulous side secreted by the endothelial cells after birth, justifying the increase of thickness to 8–12 μm in adulthood.

A specificity of the Descemet's membrane is the presence of types IV, V, VI, and VIII collagen, all arranged in an ordered structure.

4.3.5 The Endothelium

It is the layer at the back end of the cornea, in direct contact with the aqueous humor and limited at the front by the Descemet's membrane.

It is made up of a unique layer of flat, even, and hexagonal cells, which are 5–6-μm high, 15–20-μm wide, and not thicker than 6 μm. These cells have a hexagonal shape doting them with a honeycombed arrangement. The endothelial cells have almost no partition capacity; therefore, their number depends on their function. A corneal transplant requires 2,000 endothelial cells/mm² at least in order to obtain a good transparency.

These cells derive from the neural crests and then probably have the same weak partition capacity as the nervous cells (Figs. 4.7 and 4.8).

These cells have three functions: synthesis, inner barrier, and active transport necessary to the properties of corneal deturgescence. Their nucleus is big and their cytoplasm rich in organelles showing the metabolic activity (mitochondria, Golgi's apparatus, and numerous vacuoles and small granules at the apical level). The cytoplasmic membrane, to be found on the apical side of the endothelium, touches the aqueous humor. Some short microvillosities increase the surface of the membrane touching the aqueous humor. Some apical prolongations on the edge fill in the empty intercellular spaces. Some apical intercellular junctions form a discontinuous barrier permeable to the migration of small molecules from the inner chamber to the intercellular spaces. At last, there are some ciliated structures. The lateral side of the cytoplasmic membrane supports the main intercellular junctions. The basal side has a tortuous outline, which increases the contact surface with the neighboring cells.

4.3.6 The Limbus

Located on the edge of the transparent cornea, it maintains the junction with the opaque sclera. On the level of the epithelium, it is the transition between a multilayer scale-like corneal epithelium and a cylindrical conjunctival epithelium with two cellular bases, with continuity of the basement membranes. At the epithelial level, the cells of the corneal epithelium are gradually replaced by a conjunctival epithelium made of two layers of cylindrical cells accompanied by calyciform cells.

Located in the limbal epithelium, the basal cells act as stem cells for the basal cells of the corneal epithelium (Fig. 4.9).

Some melanocytes and Langerhans cells penetrate between the limbal epithelial cells. The subepithelial level

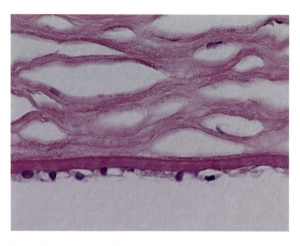

Fig. 4.7 Endothelial cells in adulthood 1

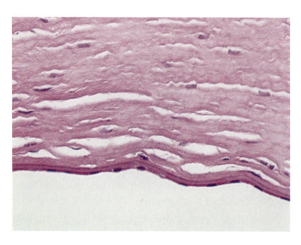

Fig. 4.8 Endothelial cells in adulthood 2

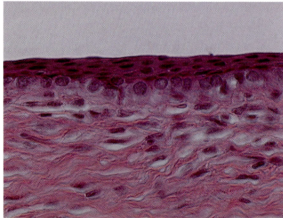

Fig. 4.9 View of the cornea at the fourth month of pregnancy: the limbal epithelium is already made of multiple layers; the basal cells set deeper are brighter and more spherical

only exists in the outer two thirds of the limbus and corresponds to the surgical limbus. It is formed by the fusion of conjunctival entities coming from the conjunctival chorion, of the Tenon's capsule and of the episclera.

The deep level is the transition between the well-organized conjunctival tissue of the stroma and the more unorganized and more cellular scleral tissue.

On this level, the collagen fibers change their orientation and lose the uniformity of size and interspace that are specific to the stroma. The cellularity increases (fibroblast, macrophages, lymphocytes, plasmocytes, melanocytes, Langerhans cells). The Descemet's membrane disappears.

The flat endothelial cells of the scleral trabeculum succeed to the corneal endothelium.

4.4 Vascularization

In normal state, the cornea has no vascularity. After lesions, scarring and the modification of the physiological conditions cause a vascularization with diminution of the corneal transparency.

4.5 Innervation

The cornea is one of the most innervated zones of the body, the discomfort or pain caused by the introduction into it of some dust or of an eyelash is a good illustration.

The amyelinic nervous fibers are to be found in the corneal stroma and also in the superficial epithelium, which is a noticeable ocular specificity. The nervous endings are to be found unconnected between the cells of the superficial epithelium and react with any contact, with chemical aggressions, with drought…

4.6 Factors of the Corneal Transparency

Transparency [5] is the essential property of the cornea because it enables the light rays to penetrate into the inside of the eye. It only starts to develop in the fourth month of fetal life until it is complete in the 6th month. Endangered in case of a severe eye burn, this critical function depends on different factors.

4.6.1 The Collagen Structure

Its arrangement in even and regular fibrillae, parallel to each other, is a fundamental element of the corneal transparency.

4.6.2 The Proteoglycans Function

They keep the interspace between fibrillae constant and act as electrostatic tampons between these fibrillae.

4.6.3 The Absence of Vascularization

In normal state, the cornea would be a too compact tissue for the vessels to penetrate it.

4.6.4 The Scarcity of Cells in the Stroma

There are various theories trying to explain the corneal transparency. According to Maurice, the transparency is due to the anatomic organization of the stroma. Indeed the collagen fibrillae, being evenly arranged and separated by constant intervals smaller than half of the wavelength, let the light rays in without any interaction.

According to Goldman and Benedek, the transparency is due to the collagen fibrillae being smaller than the light wavelength so that there is no phenomenon of diffusion.

4.6.5 The Regulation of the Hydration

The normal cornea contains 75–80% of water, with a 3.4 ratio weight of water in the stroma/dry weight. In physiological conditions, the cornea must permanently fight against hydric imbibition in order to maintain a constant thickness and keep its transparency. It is said to be in a state of deturgescence.

In this action of active deturgescence, the epithelium plays a trivial part but its function as a pump reduces the evaporation and diminishes the absorption of fluids from the tears.

Concerning the stroma, two entities are essential in the corneal hydration. On one hand, its hydrophilia can be explained by the glycosaminoglycans. Unlike these, the collagen fibrillae cannot fix water, but their parallel arrangement facilitates the expansion of the hyper-hydrated glycosaminoglycans, resulting in wide blanks without fibrillae and thus in the origin of optic modifications.

On the other hand, the cornea is located between two hypertonic grounds: tears and the aqueous humor. The rules of osmotic balance are a good explanation for the passive move of water toward the front and back sides of the cornea, so contributing in the maintenance of the relative dehydration of the stroma.

The osmolarity of a healthy human cornea should be 300 mosmol/L. Studied on 100 healthy pig corneas; more recent measurements give an osmolarity of 329 ± 61 mosmol/L [6].

We will see in Chap. 5, Physiopathology of the cornea and physiopathology of eye burns, that this corneal osmolarity must be considered as part of the immediate treatment of chemical burns. Moreover, we know that the osmolarity of a burnt cornea increases [6]. Thus, in this situation and differently to hypertonic products, the application of an iso- or hypotonic wash liquid (in comparison with a healthy cornea) like water or physiological saline onto the cornea will lead to an afflux of water into the cornea and facilitate the penetration of corrosives into the deep layers of the cornea.

At last, thanks to its function as pump, the endothelium plays a fundamental part in the maintenance of the corneal transparency.

It is about an active mechanism depending on the Na^+-K^+-ATPase enzyme located in the lateral plasma membrane of the endothelial cells. It enables the penetration of potassium into the cell against the excretion of sodium into the aqueous humor. Then this latter becomes hypertonic in comparison with the stroma and thus drains the water. In normal conditions, the pump can adapt to the physiological needs. Actually, the moves of the sodium ion are relative to those of the bicarbonate ion (responsible for the negative polarization of the back side of the endothelial cell) and to the pH variation. And yet, the bicarbonate comes from the aqueous humor and from the intracellular transformation of carbon dioxide and water by carbonic anhydrase. All of this shows the good functioning of the pumps depends on the integrity of the plasma membrane, on the cellular energy metabolism, and on the cellular enzymatic systems.

4.6.6 Mechanism of Recovery of the Corneal Transparency in case of a Burn

4.6.6.1 The Limbus

The limbus is a very important zone when an eye burn occurs: it is the region in which concentrate the stem cells that might be destroyed by the burn.

It has been well known for a long time that the renewal of the corneal epithelium depends on the limbal stem cells. At first considered as a simple theory [7], supported by several publications [8, 14], the limbal stem cells are now commonly used in transplantation as a treatment to numerous pathologies including burns. This transplantation of limbal stem cells is one of the rare successful cases of therapeutic use of stem cells for human patients [7].

The renewal of the corneal epithelium starts with the stem cells located under the basal layer of the limbus. After a few partitions, these stem cells generate amplifying transition cells, which are differentiated epithelial cells migrating toward the center of the cornea to constitute the basal cells of the corneal epithelium. Doted of an important mitotic activity, these cells generate some daughter cells that migrate toward the surface and then become intermediate cells. Then little by little, during their migration, these last ones become hyper-differentiated superficial cells, which are unable to divide and will die or desquamate [7].

On the other hand, it was usual to consider that the ability of regeneration of the endothelium is limited. Nevertheless, a recent study shows that the presence of endothelial stem cells at the level of the deep layers of the limbus would play a part in the normal replacement of the healthy epithelium and in the mechanisms of epithelial repairing too [3, 7].

The ability of the cornea to regenerate (including endothelium and epithelium) is thus concentrated at the level of the limbus. This has clinical consequences already foreseen by Hughes as early as 1946 [7] when he made limbo-conjunctival ischemia the main forecasting sign of the chemical eye burn (check clinical considerations in Chap. 7).

4.6.6.2 The Stroma

Nevertheless, the stroma might also have some ability to regenerate the cornea. That is what the Thill and his assistant study [7] seems to demonstrate with the highlighting of a new population of repairing stem cells located inside the adult human corneal stroma. These cells might evolve toward the monocyte-macrophage specie or toward the fi broblast specie (keratocytes).

There is a parallel to draw between the Thill and assistant study and the study by Kubota and Fagerlhom [15] who have demonstrated that the importance of the initial corneal edema, resulting from a burn, is correlated to the importance of the sequelar cicatricial leukoma that causes the drop of vision. The stromal lacunae, formed by the edema, will be colonized by the keratocytes. After the resorption of the edema and at the level of these lacunae, the keratocytes form a zone of cicatricial tissue, which is the origin of the leukoma. These keratocytes also produce an unorganized network of collagen fibrillae, thus causing the drop of transparency of the cornea.

This study should be considered in relation with the Jester study [16] on rabbits. The latter suggests that the postnatal development of the corneal transparency of rabbits might be associated with the decline of the density of keratocytes, with their evolution toward resting state and with their excretion of two water soluble proteins: class 1A1 dehydrogenase aldehyde and transketolase.

At last, we must mention the essential role of vitamin C in the making by keratocytes of an unorganized network of even, uniform and parallel to each other collagen fibrillae [15]. And yet when ocular burns caused by basic aggressors occur, the ascorbic acid rate in aqueous humor remains low during the month following the burn [15].

4.6.7 Action of the Intraocular Pressure

Its action on the corneal transparency only visible in case of pathology, the part played by the intraocular pressure is to be considered separately. Indeed, the big increase of the intraocular pressure may cause a stromal edema and this might happen after a chemical eye burn with lesion at the level of the trabeculum, occurring in clinical study during the second or third following week.

References

1. Raynaud, C., Bonicel, P., Rigal, D., Kantelip, B.: Anatomie de la cornée. In: Encyclopédie Médico-Chirurgicale – Ophtalmologie, p. 7. Elsevier, Paris. 21–003–A-10, (1996)
2. Rigal, D.: La barrière épithéliale. In: Rigal, D. (ed.) L'épithélium cornéen. Rapport de la Société Française d'Ophtalmologie, pp. 49–55. Masson, Paris (1993)
3. Cintron, C.: The molecular structure of the corneal stroma in health and disease. In: Chandler, J.W., Sugar, J., Edelhauser, H.F. (eds.) External Diseases: Cornea, Conjonctiva, Sclere, Eyelids, Lacrimal System, vol. 8. Mosby, London (1994)
4. Van Trappen, L., Geboes, K., Missotten, L.: Lymphocytes and Langerhans cells in the normal human cornea. Invest Ophthalmol Vis Sci **26**, 220–225 (1985)
5. Rigal-Verneil, D., Paul-Buclon, C., Sampoux, Ph.: Physiologie de la cornée. In: Encyclopédie Médico-Chirurgicale – Ophtalmologie, p. 9. Editions Techniques, Paris, 21020-C-10 (1990).
6. Berman, M., Manseau, E., Law, M., Aiken, D.: Ulceration is correlated with degradation of fibrin and fibronectin at the corneal surface. Invest Ophthalmol Vis Sci **24**, 1358–1366 (1983)
7. Mcgowan, S.L., Edelhauser, H.F., Pfister, R.R., Whikehart, D.R.: Stem cell markers in the human posterior limbus and corneal endothelium ok unwounded and wounded corneas. Mol Vis **13**, 1984–2000 (2007)
8. Thoft, R.A., Friend, J.: The X, Y, Z hypothesis of corneal epithelial maintenance. Invest Ophthalmol Vis Sci **24**, 1442–1443 (1983)
9. Kaye, D.B.: Epithelial response in penetrating keratoplasty. Am J Ophthalmol **89**, 381 (1980)
10. Davanger, M., Evensen, A.: Rôle of the pericorneal papillary structure in renewal of corneal epithelium. Nature **229**, 560–561 (1971)
11. Kinoshita, S., Friend, J., Thoft, R.A.: Sex chromatin of donor corneal epithelium in rabbits. Invest Ophthalmol Vis Sci **21**, 434–441 (1981)
12. Buck, R.C.: Measurement of centripetal migration of normal corneal epithelial cells in the mouse. Invest Ophthalmol Vis Sci **26**, 1296–1299 (1985)
13. Cotsarelis, G., Cheng, S.Z., Dong, G., Sun, T.T., Lavker, R.M.: Existence of slow-cycling limbal epithelial basal cells that can be preferentially stimulated to proliferate: implications on epithelial stem cells. Cell **57**, 201–209 (1989)
14. Chaloin-Dufau, C., Sun, T.T., Dhouailly, D.: Appearance of the keratin pair K3/K12 during embryonic and adult epithelial differentiation in the chicken and in the rabbit. Cell Differ Develop **32**, 97–108 (1990)
15. Kubota, M., Fagerholm, P.: Corneal alkali burn in the rabbit. Waterbalance, healing and transparency. Acta Ophthalmologica **69**, 635–640 (1991)
16. Jester, J.V., Ling, J., Harbell, J.: Measuring depth of injury (DOI) in an isolated rabbit eye irritation test (IRE) using biomarkers of cell death and viability. Toxicol In Vitro **24**(2), 597–604 (2010). Epub 2009 Oct 24

Physiopathology of the Cornea and Physiopathology of Eye Burns

Norbert Schrage

5.1 Physiology of the Cornea

5.1.1 Eye Burns Physiological Barriers

The barriers of the eye differ from that of skin in dimensions and mucosal organization: there are epithelial cellular barriers made of lipid layers on the eye and dry surfaces made of proteins in the stratified surfaces of the skin. Skin is protected by a superficial outer fatty film, the *stratum corneum*, and covered by a thick layer of cells, the basal cellular layer. Thanks to these thick layers, skin has a high resistance to initial diffusion of aqueous fluids and less resistance to lipophilic solvents and to acids. The initial chemical cracking of the lipid layer allows fluids to invade deeper layers of the skin. The basal cell layer and the hair follicles contain stem cells capable of epithelial regeneration.

The construction of the eye is completely different. *The outer layer* of this mucosa consists of a tiny tear layer of lipids and water which covers a superficial epithelium closed by double layer lipid membranes of 30–70 nm size interconnected by tight junctions. Three to seven layers of epithelial cells cover the stromal structures of conjunctiva or cornea. The conjunctival surface has interposed cells secreting small amounts of mucin, the so-called goblet cells, which are typically missing within the corneal epithelium. The regeneration of epithelial structures is due to the limbal stem cells located deep in the Vogt's crypts, for the cornea, and to the conjunctival stem cells lying deep in the fornices, for the conjunctiva.

The stroma of cornea and conjunctiva consists of connective tissue, which in the conjunctiva is extremely soft, containing superficial and deep vessels on the sclera located in arterial and venous vessels.

These vessels end in arcade-like structures at the limbus. The corneal stroma is made of three different main layers that differ in density of collagen and type of packing. The Bowman's membrane of the anterior stroma is part of the basal membrane of the corneal epithelium and accounts for 5% of the thickness of the central 500–600 μm cornea. The corneal stroma consists of highly ordered, horizontally organized and noninterconnected collagen I and X fibrillae that are kept in a hydrated state with a water content of 72–78% and an osmolarity of 420 mOsmol/kg [1].

The inner layer of the corneal stroma is a dense membrane of collagen like the basal membrane of the monolayer of corneal endothelium. Descemets membrane is transparent with a thickness varying from 7 to 20 μm, according to the age of the individual. Conjunctiva and cornea host nerve endings of high density in the superficial and basal layers. The cornea at the limbus smoothly changes to sclera with interconnected nontransparent collagen fibrils.

5.1.2 Physiological Mechanisms of Decontamination on the Eye

In case of surface contact of fluids with skin, typically nondefatted skin will pearl off the liquids immediately. Defatted skin tends to allow better contact for fluids. The application of soaps or detergents would lessen this initial effect. In contrast to that, the miscibility of

---

N. Schrage (✉)
Head of the Department Professorship at the RWTH Aachen, Foundator of ACTO (Aachen Center of Technology Transfer in Ophthalmology), Department of Ophthalmology of the City Hospital, Augenklinik Köln Merheim, Cologne, Germany
e-mail: schrage@acto.de

tear film with fluids is extremely high. Only slight changes of the tear film due to detergents, low alkaline or acidic solutions, cause such a distortion to the tear film that the corneal surface is altered and the feeling of scratching, itching, and pain starts. In the superficial cornea, free nerve endings detect variations in osmolarity, temperature, and homogeneity of the tear film [2]. Thus the reflex of blinking is started as an outstanding mechanical cleaning of the corneal surface. Immediate combined reflexes are tearing and vasodilatation in the conjunctiva. This effect is an early reaction of combined nerve action and, in case of tissue damage, the release of prostaglandins from damaged cells. In severe cases of exposure, a lid cramp results intentionally to squeeze out excess fluids from the corneal surface. The volume of tears increases from 10 μL/min up to 0.5 mL/min. The vasodilatation and possible opening of the fenestrated capillaries result in a strong conjunctival edema that supplies additional fluid to the tissue with increased buffering capacity. The susceptibility of this system is due to free nerve endings that are directly located under the outer layers of the corneal epithelium. Thus, only small changes in osmolarity of the tear film (drying, diving, eye drops caused itching) and change of temperature and chemical composition of the tear film result in discomfort.

Lid action efficiently removes small-sized fluids and particles from the surface without damaging it. Only particles that are captured below the lids cause mechanical irritation of the corneal surface. Under normal conditions, lid action guarantees that a double layered well-organized tear film covers the whole conjunctiva and cornea. Lid action is directly connected with a high-speed neural basic channel and the blinking reflexes may be started by mechanical touch, temperature change, or perception of objects targeting the eye. In this last case, the limitation of the system is a reaction time of about 3 ms. This is sometimes too slow to protect the eye from high-speed flying substances like high-pressure beam, splashes, particles from welding, and others. In such a situation of system failure, substances may be trapped by lid cramp within the conjunctival sac.

Substances that guarantee the chemical and mechanical stability of the cornea are mostly collagen type I and X that are mainly made of proline and hydroxyproline. Other substances that are present in a considerable amount are proteins (pK between 5.3 and 9), vitamin C (pK = 4.2), bicarbonate, glutathione, and lactate. (For more details about pK refer to Chap. 3, Sect. 3.2.4.1)

The protein buffer is a combination of all proteins that are amphoteric like their ground substance, the amino acids. Under physiological pH, we find the carboxylic acid groups as well as acidic groups and carboxylates. Thus buffering capacity is maintained. It is the same with amino groups which are present as protonized and nonprotonized. Thus both amino groups and carboxyl groups act as real amphoteric components in the living tissue. Within the cornea, the collagen is the main constituent consisting of proline (pK_1: 1.99; pK_2: 10.60), hydroxyproline, and glycine (pK_1: 2.34; pK_2: 9.6). The acid–base reaction follows the pattern below (Fig. 5.1).

The glycoproteins constituting the matrix are mainly keratin sulfate, chondroitin sulfate, and hyaluronate. The pK of the carboxyl groups on the glucuronic acid residues is 3–4, so complete ionization is present at pH 7. Those glycoproteins might act as structural buffers within the corneal tissue. Their main task is regulation of water and ion contents in the cornea. There are almost no data available on the pK constants of those glycoproteins.

The pK of a defined corrosive is given by this relation:

Acidic force:

$$\text{Acid } pK_a + H_2O \rightleftharpoons H_3O^+ + \text{base } pK_b$$

Constituents of the aqueous humor in relation to buffer capacity is shown in Fig. 5.2 and decontamination

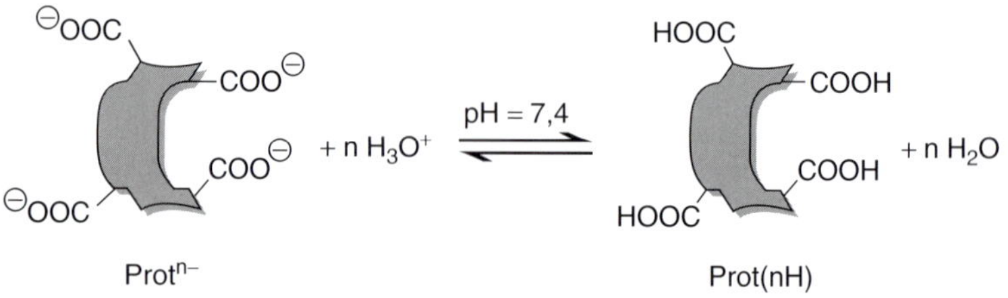

$$pH = pK_{a_{moy}} + \log \frac{[Prot^{n-}]}{[Prot(nH)]}$$

Fig. 5.1 The acid-base reaction (image from wikipedia)

5.1 Physiology of the Cornea

Fig. 5.2 Constituents of the aqueous humor in relation to buffer capacity

Alkali	pK_a	Formula	pK_a
Alkaline very strong	−10	$HClO_4$ ClO_4^-	24
Very weak	−10	HI I$^-$	24
	−6	HCl Cl$^-$	20
	−3	H_2SO_4 HSO_4^-	17
Strong	−1.74	$H_3O^+H_2O$	15.74
	−1.32	HNO_3 NO_3^-	5.32
	1.92	HSO_4^- SO_4^{2-}	2.08
Weak	2.13	H_3PO_4 $H_2PO_4^-$	11.87
	2.22	$[Fe(H_4O)_6]^{3+}$ $[Fe(OH)(H_2O)_5]^{2+}$	11.78
	3.14	HF F$^-$	10.68
	3.75	HCOOH HCOO$^-$	10.25
	4.75	CH_3COOH CH_3COO^-	9,25
	4.85	$[Al(H_2O)_6]^{3+}$ $[Al(OH)(H_2O)_5]^{2+}$	9.15
Medium strong	6.52	H_2CO_3 HCO_3^-	7.48
	6.92	H_2S HS^-	7.08
	7.20	$H_2PO_4^-$ HPO_4^{2-}	6.80
Weak	9.25	NH_4^+ NH_3	4.75
	9.40	HCN CN$^-$	4.60
	10.40	CO_3^{2-}	3.60
Strong	12.36	HPO_4^{2-} PO_4^{2-}	1.64
	13.00	HS^- S^{2-}	1.00
	15.74	H_2O OH^-	−1.74
	15.90	CH_3CH_2-OH $CH_3-CH_2-O^-$	−1.90
Very weak	23	NH_3 NH_2^-	−9
	34	CH_4 CH_3^-	−20

Fig. 5.3 Some special concentrations of Aqueous humor constituents

Anaganic substances		Organic substances	
Bicarbonate	20.2 µmol/mL	Ascorbate	1,06 µmol/mL
Chloride	131.6 µmol/mL	Glucose	2,80 µmol/mL
Potassium	3.9 µmol/mL	Lactate	4,50 µmol/mL
Sodium	152.0 µmol/mL	Protein	13,50 µmol/mL
Phosphate	0.6 µmol/mL	Citrate	0,12 µmol/mL
H^+– Ions (pH)	ca. 7.5	Creatinine	ca. 0,04 µmol/mL

Substance	Concentration in tears
pH	7.4
Osmolality	298±10
EGF (ng/mL) *Epidermal growth factor*	0.2–0.3
TGF-β (ng/mL) *Transforming Growth Factor*	2–10
NGF (pg/mL) *Nerve growth factor*	468.3±317
SP (ng/mL) *Substance P*	157.0±73.9
IGF-1 (ng/mL) *Insulin-like growth factor 1*	0.031±0.015
PDGF (ng/mL) *Platelet-Derived Growth Factor*	0–1.33
Vitamin A (mg/mL)	0.2
Albumin (mg/mL)	0.023±0.016
Fibronectin µg/mL	21
Lactoferrin (ng/mL)	1650±150
Lysozyme (mg/mL)	2.07±0.24
SIGa (µg/mL)	1190±904

Fig. 5.4 Tear fluid constituents

5.1.3 Physiology of Local Decontamination

The first and most efficient local decontamination is done by tearing. Tear production can be increased 500-fold within seconds from 10 µL/min up to 0.5 mL/min. Tear fluid contains water, mucin, lipids, lysozyme, lactoferrin, lipocalin, lacritin, immunoglobulins, glucose, urea, sodium, and potassium (Fig. 5.4). Some of the substances in lacrymal fluid fight against bacterial infection as a part of the immune system. By means of tearing, the electrolytic contents of the composition of tears move into a serum. In case of massive tearing, tear osmolarity decreases from 350 mOsmol/kg to about 280 mOsmol/kg. In case of severe alteration of vessels, the conjunctival vessels excrete, directly from the blood, a transudate which is assumed to be part of the chemosis caused by eye burns. Moreover, some fibrin can be seen in severe and distinct eye burns as coagulation on the conjunctival and corneal surface.

All those mechanisms show high efficiency against biological enemies; but the chemical capacity is very limited to basically the bicarbonate, phosphates, and the protein buffer determined by the amino-acid buffering capacities as demonstrated in Fig. 5.8. The overall chemical capacity of the cornea is less than 3 × 10^{-3} mmol (Figs. 5.6 and 5.7). There are about 150 mmol/kg ascorbic acid and about 6 µmoL/kg glutathione, and low contents of about 3.36 mmol/kg dry weight phosphate [3], bicarbonate, and from 2 to 5 mmol/kg lactate within the cornea. The cornea has a global weight of about 5 g, so that its total buffer capacity is exhausted just in case of amounts of less than 0.05 mL highly concentrated solutions and it is the

capacity in Fig. 5.3, and also some special concentrations of constituents (modified following Caprioli 1992).

Fig. 5.5 Acidic buffering of the healthy pig cornea. There is considerable deviation of pH development from simple dilution curve with buffering within the corneal tissue

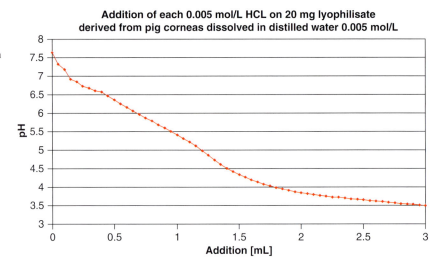

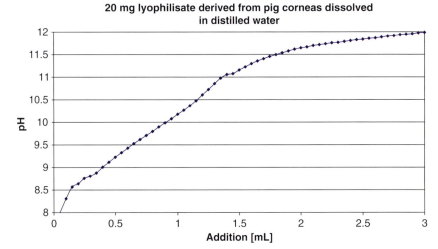

Fig. 5.6 Alkaline buffering of the corneal tissue. There is a considerable deviation of pH development from dilution curve, indicating buffering characteristics of the cornea

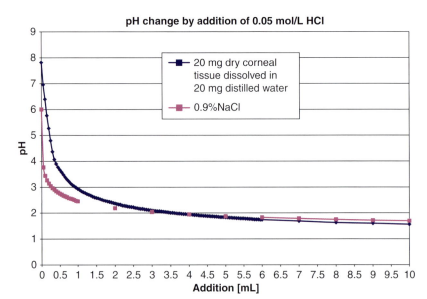

Fig. 5.7 Difference of acidic buffering of corneal tissue from dilution curve in water of the same mass. There is a considerable difference between both curves indicating buffering characteristics

case in all eye burns. Further, we might argue that there is a biological buffer within the extracellular matrix. This can be denied due to measurements performed on whole corneas as shown in Figs. 5.6 and 5.7. Thus it becomes clearer that corrosives with a mass exceeding the mass of the above-described natural buffers will cause a severe alteration of the corneal structure proteins and jeopardize the survival of this organ.

When limited to narrow borders, higher tearing and increased aqueous humor secretion are the only ways to increase the buffering capacity of the eye.

5.1.4 Limits of Physiological Decontamination

The biologically developed resistance and buffering systems are organized within the common limits of biological chemicals and toxic substances. Those substances are weak alkalis and acids from flowers and fruit, immunoreactive vasodilators of insects and animals, and peroxides from physiological light exposition. Within the human body, there is a real buffer system thanks to the bicarbonate and phosphate system. Other physiologically available buffers are amino acids which are amphoteric, and the ascorbate, glutathione, tocopherol system which guarantees a radical decontamination.

This type of buffering capacity of the cornea can be followed by microtitration of corneal homogenate, produced from 1,000 pig corneas, under continuous measurement of pH with addition of Acid (HCl) in Figs. 5.5 and 5.7 and Alkali (NaOH) in Fig. 5.6.

Most interesting about amino acids buffering, and thereby, the capacity of the protein buffer, are the narrow limits between a dissociation constant of 5.3 to 9. Thus, the exceeding of the buffering capacity from amino acids on higher or lower pHs, as the mentioned limits of 5.3–9, result in an immediate stop of biochemical activity such as protein biosynthesis by protonization or deprotonization of the amino acid molecule. Here, we face a fundamental limitation of metabolic activity within the cellular turnover. The dissociation constants, especially those of the amino acids, are crucial in the definition of the pH level at which amino acids do not react any longer as real amphoteres. To give more insight into this, we graphically work up the amino acid pK dissociation constants within a sketch presented under Fig. 5.8.

The survival depends on the availability of ions that define the electronegativity and the ion force of the cellular compartment. Moreover, specific ions such as Zn, Fe, and Ca are essential for enzymatic activity. Different types of specific burns or intoxications result in severe damages with a relatively low immediate visibility of the occurred distortions. This is a typical pattern of HF burns that chelate all calcium and magnesium

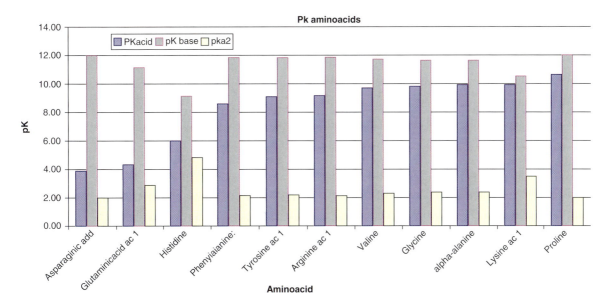

Fig. 5.8 pKa and b of amino acids. The excess of pH from limits within two of these constants results in loss of bio availability of the compound for protein biosynthesis due to complete protonization of the compound

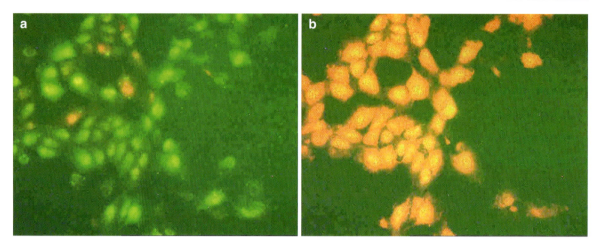

Fig. 5.9 (a) Cells before exposure and (b) cells 30 s after exposure to HF

from cells: Calcein with Ca^{2+} loaded (*green*) and calcein depleted from Ca^{2+} (*red*) are shown. Calcein or fluorescein complex is used as indicator of complexion for calcium ion with EDTA. Exposure of fibroblasts in cell culture toward a 0.0002% HF solution is shown in Fig. 5.9a and b. Excitation and emission wavelengths are 495/515 nm. Fluorometric possibilities are shown on orange color crystals. The green cells turn to red by complete depletion of free calcium from the cellular body.

This is similar to the highly selective action of oxygen removal from Fe^{++} by means of CO (carbon monoxide) or the intoxication of the metabolic breathing by CN^- (cyanide ion). All these specific types of intoxications systemically result in ceasing of local metabolic activity with consecutive cellular necrosis.

Glutathione in reduced (GSH) and oxidized form (GSSG) ratios given within the cornea before and after exposure to oxidative stress is shown in Fig. 5.10.

A real confirmation that chemical reaction dependent on proteinic pKa is a real mechanism that takes place during the time course of eye burn has been presented by Gerard et al. [4]. They found a time-dependent and stepwise increase of the pH within the cornea after eye burn with ammonia.

This indicates the probability of levels of reactions because of the different pKa of ammonia and the presence in the cornea of substances producing a stepwise reaction from lower to higher pKa.

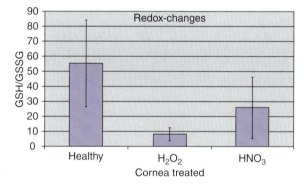

Fig. 5.10 GHS/GSSG ration before and after oxidative stress

5.1.5 Limits between Irritation and Burn

Our body is used to repair small accidents of mechanical or chemical origin. These accidents of biological origin are due to stinging by nettles or insects on eye and skin. Further, there are mechanical damages that are used to be repaired within a short time – as seen in the *ex vivo* eye irritation test (EVEIT) – such as the healing of mechanical damage *ex vivo* within a short period of 3 days observed on the isolated rabbit cornea (Fig. 5.11a and b).

The damage is healed by highly regenerative cellular structures on surfaces that are sustained by depots of stem cells that react by reproducing the required cells by means of increased dividing rate and metabolic

5.2 Pathophysiology of Eye Burns

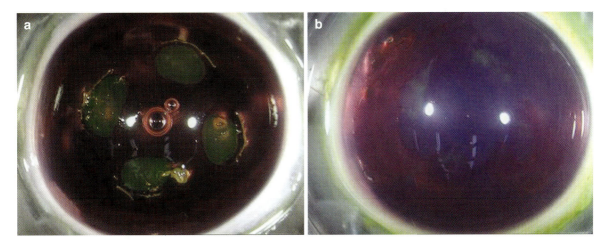

Fig. 5.11 (**a**) Abrasion at start of the experiment and (**b**) healed abrasion at day 4

activity. Called irritation, this process is due to an increased release of vasoactive substances, proinflammatory mediators such as IL-8 (Interleukin) and VEGF (Vascular endothelial growth factor). These mechanisms offer the possibility of cleavage of wounds, removal of necrosis, and installation of healing tissues. This temporarily increased biochemical activity is regulated and is stopped by inhibitors of inflammation released from closed cellular epithelium when healing is achieved. The result of an irritation is a healing "*ad integrum.*" In contrast to this, burns are defined as a trauma that is not self limiting. Thus additional measures such as medical wound cleavage, a surgical removal of necrosis, and an initiation of healing must be done. Furthermore, an efficient modification of the inflammation is required by means of steroids and nonsteroidal compounds. Only under these circumstances, healing or regulated scar formation can be achieved.

5.1.6 Eye Burns

Eye burns are a process that develops during a chemical or thermal exposure that is of exceeding mass, contact time, chemical reactivity, and temperature until the exhaustion of the protective mechanisms of the eye. The most plastic description of this process can be given in images that are obtained by optical coherence tomography [5].

Figure 5.12a shows the impregnation of a cornea with 1 mol NaOH over the time of exposure. In Fig. 5.12b, image shows the impregnation speed for some 2 mol NaOH. There is a considerably higher invasion speed of the corrosive depending on concentration over time. Thus the integral of concentration over time gives an answer to limits between irritation and burn.

The disease of burn is characterized by an overwhelming inflammation, with invasion of leucocytes within the whole tissue without any modulation of tissue breakdown, and an ulceration of the necrotic tissues.

Delayed intervention results in much more severe damage to the eye [6].

5.2 Pathophysiology of Eye Burns[1]

5.2.1 Types of Burns and Eye Irritation

The expressions of eye irritation and eye burns define a variety of interactions of chemical fluids, powders, and foreign bodies when they interfere with the ocular surface [7]. In this chapter, we shall focus on the mechanistic understanding of the known facts in this field.

---

[1]Dedicated to the 75th anniversary of Prof. Dr. med. M. Reim, a great researcher and teacher in Ophthalmology and especially in the research and clinical work on eye burns.

Fig. 5.12 (**a**) Impregnation speed of a cornea with 1 mol NaOH and (**b**) impregnation speed of a cornea with 2 mol NaOH

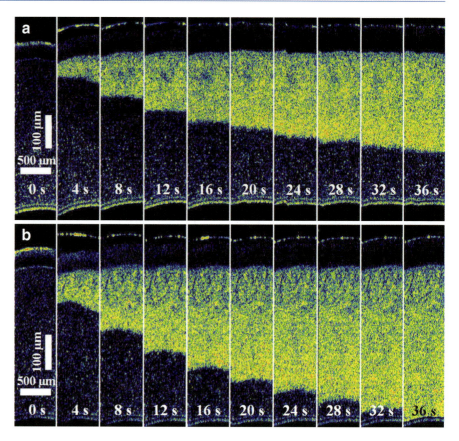

The most important knowledge in this field is to be found in experiments that have been performed within the last 20 years in a systematic approach on explaining circumstances of eye burns, systematic evaluation of types of corrosives, and the evaluation of corrosives in organotypic experiments.

The newer efforts of the European community with the REACH initiative and the prohibition of animal experiments for the allowance of cosmetics lead to a new systematic approach on the understanding of the mechanisms of eye irritation and the related eye burns.

In clinical understanding, we find typical and different patterns of eye irritations and eye burns. The origin of all clinical appearance is always related to damage to the structure as known from strong alkali and strong acids. There are also specific interactions with loss of calcium in case of fluoride ions leading to a complete stop of cellular life within seconds to not yet well-defined interactions of peroxides and oxygen radicals with membranes, leading especially to proinflammatory cellular response. Other types of eye burns relate to membrane active irritants as typically known from detergents of different types like anionic, cationic, and nonionic [8]. Severe burns also result from other substances (such as reducing agents, alkylating agents, solvents, ionizing chemicals, etc.) that are mostly known from accidents in heuristic cases and case collections of clinical treatment [9].

5.2.2 Mechanisms of Corneal Burns

5.2.2.1 Contact Mechanisms

The first contact of a corrosive with the eye surface is normally with the skin when eyes are closed and the propagation of the corrosive into the tear fluid is done by lipid transport from the skin surface into the tear film well known as from the inner lid angle and about 2 mm zone out of the lid margin. Other mechanisms of delivery to the eye itself are smearing from fingers, direct projections such as drop-like splashes and shallowing of low pressure or "bathing" to beams of high pressure as typically known from opening of tubings with high hydrostatic pressure, pumping stations, or pressure delivery of fluids. In some cases, a mechanical trauma is added to the corrosive delivery, especially in cases of exploding accumulators or exploding tubings or connectors of concrete pumps. We and many others have observed that, beside a severe trauma of the anterior segment, an additional chemical [10] and blunt trauma [11] to the retina and elevated intraocular pressure directly after the initial trauma [12] can be decisive for the visual outcome.

5.2.2.2 Thermal Contact

Particles

The well-known mechanism of surface contact of hot devices like curling iron [13] and particles relates to heat, thermal conductivity, and time of contact. It is a common fact that the higher the temperature difference and the higher the thermal conductivity, the more the tissue damage. Typically, thermal eye burns, such as those caused by a single touch with a curling iron, are not too harmful, as described below [13]. But, like it happens in about 20% of all cases, if hot chemicals touch the eye, damage is more severe. Damage from small iron particles from iron cutting or welding occur frequently and give rust scars in the cornea which might impair vision when centrally located [14]. Most chemicals are delivered to the eye at temperatures of the surroundings. Cold and frozen particles transfer heat from the body to the particle and lead to freezing damage limited by water thermal conductivity, freezing point, and vascular reserve of the damaged tissue [15].

Hot Fluids

Hot fluids follow the mechanism of the thermodynamic speeding up of any reaction due to faster diffusion and higher reactivity in water-containing surrounding. The limits of water-containing fluids and their chemical interaction are relative to the freezing and the boiling points of the resulting mixtures of corrosive and tissue fluids. Therefore, in highly dissociated corrosives, the freezing point depression acts to temperatures up to −40°C. In any case of chemical fluid contact, we state that the higher the temperature of immediate contact is, the bigger the expected damage is.

Steam

In case of a steam delivery, the initial reaction and interaction with the ocular tissue result in a strong heat transfer by means of transfer of the condensation energy into the tissue. To get an idea of the amount of energy delivered to the tissue by this, we have to face that condensation gives the same amount of energy needed to boil up water from 20°C to 100°C. Most of the times the reflexive lid closure prevents the inner eye with conjunctiva and cornea from severe damage, and the type of burn that occurs most often is a lid angle surface coagulation with full recovery.

Liquid Metals

Liquid metal burns are known as projections from blast furnace tap or the situation of loading with delivery of bulk into liquid metal. Metal is normally of low viscosity like water and spreads on skin and eye. Thus projections of liquid metal do not behave like viscous materials but like water and spread their enormous heat onto wide areas. When eventually cooling down, liquid metal is trapped in the conjunctival sac. When this happens, there is a maximum heat transfer with high thermoconductivity from metallic surfaces to the conjunctiva with immediate water evaporation and consecutive heat transfer from the metal to the eye up to carbonization of the tissues [16, 17].

Cold Gazes

Further, heat transfers like cold delivery of liquid gazes mostly do not harm too much because of the Leyden frost phenomenon of limited heat transfer in any region of immediate low heat conductivity with evaporation of liquid gazes. Cold metals transfer heat from the conjunctival surfaces within seconds and cold burns are a very uncommon accidental mechanism, but often found in case of medical treatments of the eye [18].

5.2.2.3 Eye Burns with Chemically Active Foreign Bodies

Different foreign body burns may act and develop differently. First are insoluble but chemically reactive foreign bodies that are subject of the typical iron-containing foreign body touching the eye in all types of metal processing professions. The process is an initial mechanical attachment of a hot and high surface metallic foreign body to the corneal or conjunctival surface. Next, an ionic dissolving of iron from the surface of the particle and under oxygen exposure on the eye surface leads to the formation of rust [19] that moves into the tissue and forms the typical aspect around the particles. This process might, if removal is delayed, result in complete dissolving of the particle and severe inflammation triggered by iron oxide [20].

Another foreign body that typically interferes in eye burns is calcium oxide in any form like fluid concrete to fresh mixtures of CaO (Calcium oxide) with water. The reactive CaO dissolves with the water being attracted from the eye into Ca^{++} with additional hydroxyl ions. The saponification of the tissues by the alkali results in the diffusion of the foreign body into the tissue with deep corneal foreign body, difficult to remove [21]. All other known bioactive foreign bodies usually, more or less, follow these two different reaction types.

5.2.2.4 Eye Burns with Chemically Reactive Fluids

Alkali

Alkali is a frequent cause of eye burns as again confirmed in a recent study of Midelfarth [22]. Alkali reacts with the tissue surface by concentration and time-dependent dissolution of the lipid membranes of epithelial cells; the chemical mechanism is saponification of lipids with loss of all membranous barriers. Lipid saponification of membranous lipids starts at a pH over 11 [23].

The penetration into the tissue follows the initial breakdown of the epithelial barrier. This results in an immediate and strong edema of the conjunctiva, known as chemosis, due to a water influx from the surrounding tissue, vascular leakage, tears, and applied fluids. The cornea itself loads up with ions to a measured osmolarity of 1,830 mOsmol/kg after a 1 mol NaOH burn for 30 s [24]. The penetration of strong alkali has been systematically tested on sodium hydroxide by means of evaluation of the anterior chamber pH. This pH change typically occurs within 2 min after exposure of the corneal surface. The change of the cornea shows immediate swelling of the corneal tissue in an order of magnitude of 20%, as published by Kompa et al in 2000. Increasing opacity of the cornea is a result of the tissue edema and of the change of the fibrillary structure of the collagen.

Acids

Acids act on the organic tissues when in a range of pH under 5. The free hydrogen ion is highly reactive and causes severe coagulation of proteins with superficial and deep ulceration if the excess of acid is high enough. The propagation of acids into the tissue is less fast than that of alkali. In case of hydro sulfuric acid, we found very fast propagation of the acid into the anterior chamber. We believe that in highly concentrated acids, the shrinkage of the tissue allows faster diffusion [25].

Peroxides

Peroxides react by free electron transfer from one molecule to the next. This gives typically slower damage characteristics. The body is quite used to decontaminate free radicals by means of the superoxide dismutase [26]; the system consists of glutathione, tocopherol, and ascorbic acid with its regeneration by means of the glutathione peroxidase. Further, the enzyme catalase is highly reactive toward hydrogen peroxide and its decontamination [27]. If this system is exhausted, the damage of any chemical structure results in membrane lysis, DNA strain breaks, and protein damage; this causes a delayed onset of necrosis which is commonly known on the eye of contact lens wearers forgetting to neutralize their 3% hydrogen peroxide containing cleaning solutions. The onset of symptoms is late, from 6 h to 3 days after exposure, being proven by Maurer et al. [28] in their experimental exposure on rabbits (Fig. 5.13).

Sometimes severe damage of the cornea can occur [29, 30]. The conjunctival damage is mostly low due to the good vascularization and fast repair by means of blood refilling of the protective mechanisms.

We found severe endothelial and stromal damage after exposure to hydrogen peroxide with a defined 10 μL exposure of a 7 mm diameter on the cornea in the EVEIT model. These exposures lead in all cases to a dose-dependent endothelial dysmorphy in lower

5.2 Pathophysiology of Eye Burns

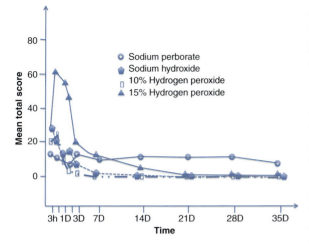

Fig. 5.13 Corneal exposure to peroxides

concentrations and to endothelial necrosis in higher concentrations. The severity of the damage can be judged by the epithelial necrosis with a nonhealing corneal erosion in the EVEIT model (Fig. 5.14).

Endothelial defects of *ex vivo* corneas at different time points after exposure to various concentrations of H_2O_2 are shown in Fig. 5.15. The ordinate shows the score of epithelial defects. The bars over the abscissa give the mean values and standard deviations, from left to right with exposure to 1.5, 3, 6, and 12% H_2O_2, respectively, for each concentration of H_2O_2. The time points zero mark the state immediately after application of H_2O_2, then the healing progress or failure on day 2 and 7 is presented. Each bar represents the mean value of $n = 3$ individual *ex vivo* corneas; no dose responses, but increasing damage with time.

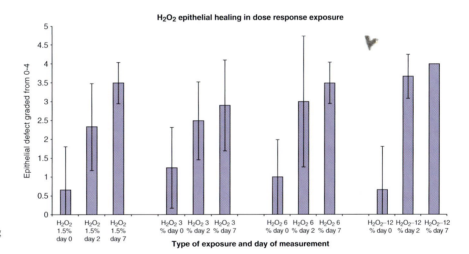

Fig. 5.14 Epithelial healing after exposure to H_2O_2

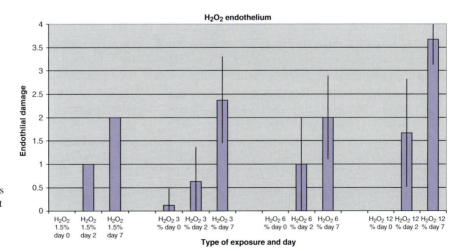

Fig. 5.15 Endothelial defects of *ex vivo* corneas at different time points after exposure to various concentrations of H_2O_2

Damage to the endothelium of *ex vivo* corneas after exposure of the epithelial surface to 1.5, 3.0, 6.0, and 12.0% H_2O_2 is shown (Fig. 5.15). The ordinate shows the endothelial damage score. The bars over the abscissa refer to the score on days 2 and 7, with the concentrations applied, respectively. Each of the bars over 1.5, 6.0, and 12.0% H_2O_2 represents $n = 3$ experiments. With 3% H_2O_2 the endothelia of $n = 8$ experiments were evaluated. Endothelial damage on day 2 shows a clear dose response.

There is a slight inhomogeneity concerning the dose response within the graphs, which is related to the difficulty to deliver the hydrogen peroxide to the tissue by means of catalase that is present within epithelial cells resulting in immediate "bubbling." Therefore only the low and very high concentrations differ significantly.

Hydrofluoric Acid

HF is an acid with low dissociation potential and does not mostly react as an acid but primarily does with divalent cations like Mg^{++} or Ca^{++}. This reaction results in fluorspar and calcspar. These highly insoluble materials precipitate within the tissue and, when the fluor reacts, the hydrogen ion is released and by dissociation new ions are released from the low dissociated fluid. This mechanism explains the high corrosivity and the deep tissue action of this type of burn. There is up to now little clinical experience on eye burns with specific decontamination drugs like calcium gluconate which is argued to be toxic in case of subconjunctival injection of 1% [31]. In current literature, there was a controversial discussion as to whether or not a washing with Hexafluorine® is useful or not. In experiments on rat skin, there were differing results between two different groups trying similar treatments [32]. The reality of the clinical use is different following the case report series presented by Mathieu et al. [33], Söderberg et al. [34], and Hall et al. [35]. The clinical question is solved by a lot of case reports with successful clinical treatment with this substance and with current experimental results on the eye. There is a considerable knowledge in recent literature showing that, in direct comparison of similar eye burns with HF, the Hexafluorine® decontamination gives the clearest tissue and the lowest penetration of HF into the corneal tissue [36].

Detergents/Solvents

Long-term exposures to detergents were found to be harmful to the ocular surface. This might be correlated to the early lysis of cellular structures and thereby, the enhanced diffusion into the deeper layers of the corneal stroma. The secondary effects might be an endothelial necrosis and a corneal swelling as we observed in each of the 16 corneas in the EVEIT on rabbit corneas with Tomadol 14–5 (10%), and Tomadol 45–7 (3%). At the mentioned concentrations, these detergents completely have destroyed the corneas. This is in contrast to low toxicity of Sodium-Lauryl Sulfate but can be confirmed for Benzalkonium chloride which is of high toxicity for the eye in higher doses and repeated dosing [37].Generally, soaps tend to be not too dangerous if present in low concentrations. Higher concentrations and longer exposure times with such detergents are able to dissolute membranes of cells, and thereby can cause harm to cellular structures. The most common substance in this context is Benzalkonium chloride known for its epitheliotoxicity to the eye.

5.2.3 Influence of Osmolarity

Osmolarity is the physical result of the dissociation of substances in fluids. It can be measured by freeze point depression. The effects of osmolar changes are mostly seen on semipermeable membranes as known from almost all membranes of living tissues. The known effects on erythrocytes such as the formation of blown-up spherocytes in hypoosmolar conditions and shrinkage in hyperosmolar conditions are transferable to all other cells.

Osmolar stress is a source of dysfunction and cell destruction [38].

If powders or soluble substances are delivered onto the ocular surface they will dissolve. By this dissolving, a huge amount of ions is delivered and osmolarity of tears will result in localized osmolar stress. Ocular burn is related to the contact of highly concentrated substances of more or less dissociation onto the eye. Even a crystal of NaCl is known to be of high corrosivity and irritation due to the locally caused severe osmolar changes [39].

In experiments, we have found that the proper tissue osmolarity of the cornea is 420 mOsmol/kg [40].

After eye burns by exposure of the cornea to 1 mol NaOH for 30 s, osmolarity was 1,380 mOsmol/kg. This reflects the huge changes of osmolarity during eye burns and possibly during treatment. The rinsing with tap water results in an extreme lowering of the osmolarity into the region of 0 mOsmol/kg on the ocular surface.

In experiments in which we have used medium supply for cell cultures with 800 mOsmol/kg, we have found the cellular resistance, needed to keep cellular integrity without exploding cells, to be acutely above 280 mOsmol/kg [41]. Lower osmolarities resulted in lysis of cells. The rinsing concept of Diphoterine® with an osmolarity of 820 mOsmol/kg reflects a stepwise reduction of the osmolar constitution of the tissues [42].

5.2.4 Penetration Characteristics

In any type of ocular burn and later on rinsing therapy, we have found that the speed of the penetration was roughly correlated to the concentration of the corrosive and the type of corrosive. This question is still scientifically open but estimations of penetration of sodium hydroxide are from about 5–8 μm/s depth propagation into the tissues, derived from measurements of Rihawi et al. on rabbit corneas [43]. Theoretical work on penetration characteristics of different chemicals have been published by Pospisil and Holzhuetter [44]. They have proved that, in first order estimation, the chemical properties like molecular size and shape, partition coefficients, and the type of interaction with the intrinsic membrane parameters determine the penetration characteristics. In very good estimations, they have shown that, for a various set of test substances, the penetration is almost exactly predicted by their modelization.

5.2.5 Cellular Survival

Cellular survival is crucial for any later regeneration. The survival has to be divided into two major cell types: first the differentiated cells that can be replaced by their precursors like fibroblasts and epithelial cells deriving from stem cells, and those which cannot be replaced due to missing stem cells or missing differentiation of stem cells toward this type of cells, like the human corneal endothelium.

There are major key issues on stem cells that explain poor prognosis of Grade III burns including ischemia of the limbus to an extent of more than 50%, according to the classification of Reim [45]. The overall concept of stem cell survival on the cornea was published by Tseng [46]. This concept gives a clear insight that survival of stem cells is crucial for successful corneal reepithelialization.

This leads to one key issue in treating the corneal eye burns with the necessity of taking measures that prevent the cornea from additional damage, to prevent damage of the differentiated cells, and more to keep stem cells alive and dedifferentiated. Therefore, any measure in treatment of corneal eye burns must prevent additional damage from cells.

Damage of cells includes necrosis-like lysis of membranes, coagulation of proteins, and delivery of proinflammatory cells and mediators, and induction of programmed cell death called apoptosis. Any apoptosis-inducing factors and any differentiation-producing factors in the postburn period must be treated to prevent a late degeneration of the anterior segment. That this concept is a successful one has been shown recently at the ARVO meeting by Behrens et al. [47, 48] when treating a burnt mouse eye with amniotic fluid resulted in a complete restoration of the anterior segment after an initial opaque cornea. These results rely on a former work on the inhibition of TGF beta by amniotic fluids [49] as hint that a stem cell rescue might be essential for future action in early eye burn treatment. This must be the goal to achieve in early and late therapy concepts of eye burns. Mostly, the scientifically approved use of corticosteroids in preventing the early massive leucocytic invasion and lytic reaction [50] confirms this strategy and might be updated by more specific stem cell and neovascularization blocking agents. Corneal stromal survival is dependent on a restoration of keratocytes and the inhibition of transformation to fibroblasts due to inflammation, mediators, and severe proliferation stimulus. Endothelial survival is well known to be a fact in severe eye burns [51] and is the most outstanding circumstance to guarantee corneal survival. If a higher amount of the endothelium is damaged, only little chances on visual rehabilitation without corneal graft are given.

5.2.6 Release of Inflammatory Mediators

From clinical observations and from experimental data we know that the primary situation after eye burns results in severe release of proinflammatory mediators. These mediators start the disastrous disease that leads to loss of sight by chronic inflammation. This can be measured in vivo and *ex vivo* on Prostaglandins as showed in an eye burn model on rabbits in Fig. 5.16.

Healthy cornea (purple) and burnt corneas with 3% hydrogen peroxide (blue) and sodium hydroxide (yellow) are shown. It is completely clear that, with increasing necrosis at day 6 and 7, the NaOH-burnt cornea releases less Prostaglandin, while the still inflamed but vital cornea burnt with hydrogen peroxide releases increasing amounts of Prostaglandin J2. (Vertical red bar gives time point of exposure for 30 s).

Clinically, we address this topic by high doses of steroids and massive anti-inflammatory measures like topical steroids, cyclosporine A, and rinsing of the eye under the presumption that it would remove the mediator-rich transudates [52] that are enriched with proteolytic enzymes like the *N*-actyl-glucosaminidase. Further studies have observed high IL-8 and IL-1 rates in corneas after eye burns [53]. These data could be reproduced in the EVEIT system with IL-8 being upregulated for NaOH and also for the sodium lauryl sulfate (SLS) (Fig. 5.17) in a dose-dependent manner.

Interleukin-8 (IL-8) levels as found in the supernatant rinsing medium (SM) in the EVEIT system of *ex vivo* corneas after exposure to various concentrations of a very common detergent (soap)– sodium lauryl sulfate (SLS) – are shown. The ordinate shows IL-8 levels in % of initial values after 36 hours of perfusion, i.e., immediately before the experimental exposure. The concentrations of SLS used in each set of experiments are indicated in the abscissa. Three corneas of each were exposed to 1.5, 3.0, or 15.0% and 30.0% SLS (*n* = 3). The time scale of the analysis is explained on the right side of the diagram.

Further we have found, like described by other authors, that beside prostaglandins being upregulated depending on the type of trauma, the highly upregulated VEGF indicates a severe proinflammatory reaction and, in combination with IL-8, an induction of apoptosis [54]. The release of IL-6 and IL-8 could be suppressed by using pentoxyphylline [55]. From this observation, it was concluded, that IL-8 was produced by the regenerating corneal epithelium or keratocytes in the denuded stroma. The substance P and pain are positively correlated with the appearance of IL-8 produced by keratocytes or corneal epithelial cells. The incomplete healing is a typical pattern of progressive epithelial wounds after NaOH and H_2O_2 exposure. These patterns of epithelial regeneration are well known from clinical observation. Even the time span of epithelial closure coincides with the healing in human patients [56]. There are typical responses on the corrosive delivery including opacity of the cornea, epithelial break ups, moving erosions, and other

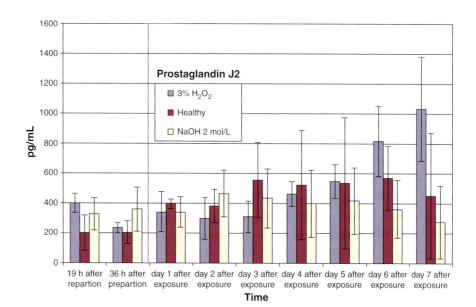

Fig. 5.16 Release of inflammatory mediators

5.2 Pathophysiology of Eye Burns

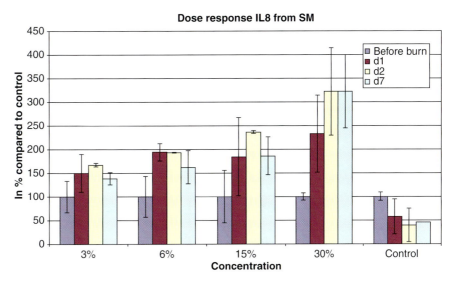

Fig. 5.17 Dose response SLS IL-8 from SM

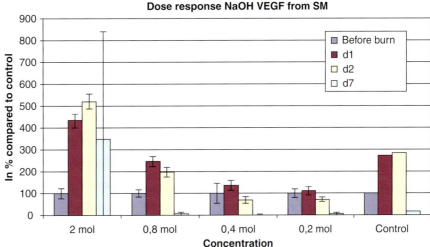

Fig. 5.18 VEGF after NaOH corneal exposure

patterns that are known from eye burn patients and seen in previous work on rabbit eyes [57]. The released VEGF (Fig. 5.18) after chemical trauma is one of the promoter factors of the severe inflammation producing healing problems after eye burns [58]. IL-1 is one factor involved in continued inflammation, promoting edema of the cornea [59].

Figure 5.18 shows vascular endothelial growth factor (VEGF) levels in the supernatant rinsing media of the epithelial side in the EVEIT system (SM) of *ex vivo* corneas after exposure to various concentrations of NaOH. The ordinate shows VEGF levels in percentage of initial values after 36 h of perfusion, i.e., immediately before the experimental exposure. The concentrations of NaOH used in each set of experiments are indicated in the abscissa. Three corneas each were exposed to 0.2, 0.4, or 0.8 mol NaOH ($n = 3$). Corneas ($n = 16$) were exposed to 2 mol NaOH. The time scale of the analysis is explained on the upper side of the diagram.

VEGF levels as found in the supernatant rinsing medium (SM) of *ex vivo* corneas after exposure to various concentrations of SLS are shown in Fig. 5.19. The ordinate shows VEGF levels in percentage of initial values after 36 h of perfusion, i.e., immediately before the experimental exposure. The concentrations of SLS used in each set of experiments are indicated in the abscissa. Three corneas each were exposed to 1.5, 3.0, or 15.0 and 30.0% SLS ($n = 3$). The time scale of the analyses is explained on the right side of the diagram.

All these measurements underline the basic effects of regulated and specific response of the biological

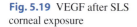

Fig. 5.19 VEGF after SLS corneal exposure

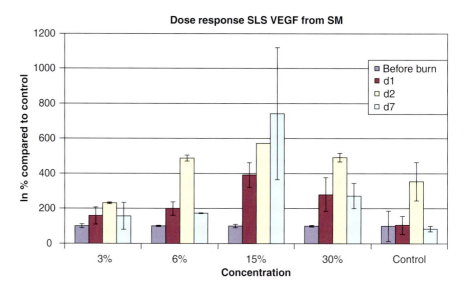

structure of the cornea toward a chemical trauma. There is a considerable difference between time points of observation, types of exposure, and specific reactions of the tissue. Due to the mediator release, the response of the whole organism is triggered. Thus, prostaglandin release will cause vascular changes, itching, and pain; substance P release gives similar reactions. The interleukins result in attraction of cells from the blood vessels, and the VEGF is a strong factor of the totally undesired vascularization of the clear cornea. We can show by these experimental data that, beyond doubt, in contrast to former assumptions, the cornea itself triggers the reaction of the surrounding tissues and that the key role of treatment is to treat the release of inflammation from the cornea.

References

1. Schrage, N.F., Flick, S., Redbrake, C., Reim, M.: Electrolytes in the cornea: a therapeutic challenge. Graefes Arch Clin Exp Ophthalmol **234**(12), 761–764 (1996)
2. Schrage, N.F., Flick, S., von Fischern, T., Wenzel, M.: Temperaturveränderungen der Hornhaut unter verschiedenen Verbänden. Ophthalmologe **94**(7), 492–495 (1997)
3. von Fischern, T., Lorenz, U., Burchard, W.-G., Reim, M., Schrage, N.F.: Changes in mineral composition of rabbit corneas after alkali burn. Graefes Arch Clin Exp Ophthalmol **1998**) **236**, 553–558 (1998)
4. Gerard, M., Louis, V., Merle, H., Josset, P., Menerath, J.M., Blomet, J.: Experimental study about intra-ocular penetration of ammonia. J Fr Ophtalmol **22**(10), 1047–1053 (1999). French
5. Spöler, F., Frentz, M., Först, M., Kurz, H., Schrage, N.F.: Dynamic analysis of chemical eye burns using high-resolution optical coherence tomography. J Biomed Opt **12**(4), 041203 (2007)
6. Rihawi, S., Frentz, M., Becker, J., Reim, M., Schrage, N.F.: The consequences of delayed intervention when treating chemical eye burns. Graefes Arch Clin Exp Ophthalmol **245**(10), 1507–1513 (2007)
7. Kuckelkorn, R., Kottek, A., Schrage, N., Reim, M.: Poor prognosis of severe chemical and thermal eye burns: the need for adequate emergency care and primary prevention. Int Arch Occup Environ Health **67**(4), 281–284 (1995)
8. Maurer, J.K., Parker, R.D., Jester, J.V.: Extent of initial corneal injury as the mechanistic basis for ocular irritation: key findings and recommendations for the development of alternative assays. Regul Toxicol Pharmacol **36**(1), 106–117 (2002)
9. Kuckelkorn, R., Makropoulos, W., Kottek, A., Reim, M.: Retrospective study of severe alkali burns of the eyes. Klin Monatsbl Augenheilkd **203**(6), 397–402 (1993)
10. Koh, H.J., Kim, S.H., Kwon, O.W.: Inadvertent topical exposure to isocyanates caused damage to the entire eyeball. Korean J Ophthalmol **14**(1), 38–40 (2000)
11. Miyamoto, F., Sotozono, C., Ikeda, T., Kinoshita, S.: Retinal cytokine response in mouse alkali-burned eye. Ophthalmic Res **30**(3), 168–171 (1998)
12. Green, K., Paterson, C.A., Siddiqui, A.: Ocular blood flow after experimental alkali burns and prostaglandin administration. Arch Ophthalmol **103**(4), 569–571 (1985)
13. Qazi, K., Gerson, L.W., Christopher, N.C., Kessler, E., Ida, N.: Curling iron-related injuries presenting to U.S. emergency departments. Acad Emerg Med **8**(4), 395–397 (2001)
14. Nicaeus, T., Erb, C., Rohrbach, M., Thiel, H.J.: An analysis of 148 outpatient treated occupational accidents. Klin Monatsbl Augenheilkd **209**(4), A7–A11 (1996)
15. Vajpayee, R.B., Gupta, N.K., Angra, S.K., Chhabra, V.K., Sandramouli, S., Kishore, K.: Contact thermal burns of the cornea. Can J Ophthalmol **26**(4), 215–218 (1991)

References

16. Pelletier, C.R., Jordan, D.R.: An unusual and severe thermal burn to the eye and adnexa. Can J Ophthalmol **31**(6), 319–323 (1996)
17. Mirza, G.E., Karakucuk, S.: A rare corneal injury caused by molten lead. Acta Ophthalmol (Copenh) **71**(4), 573–574 (1993)
18. Tuppurainen, K.: Cryotherapy for eyelid and periocular basal cell carcinomas: outcome in 166 cases over an 8-year period. Graefes Arch Clin Exp Ophthalmol **233**(4), 205–208 (1995)
19. Jayamanne, D.G., Bell, R.W.: Non-penetrating corneal foreign body injuries: factors affecting delay in rehabilitation of patients. J Accid Emerg Med **11**(3), 195–197 (1994)
20. Liston, R.L., Olson, R.J., Mamalis, N.: A comparison of rust-ring removal methods in a rabbit model: small-gauge hypodermic needle versus electric drill. Ann Ophthalmol **23**(1), 24–27 (1991)
21. Reim, M., Redbrake, C., Schrage, N.: Chemical and thermal injuries of the eyes. Surgical and medical treatment based on clinical and pathophysiological findings. Arch Soc Esp Oftalmol **76**(2), 79–124 (2001)
22. Midelfart, A., Hagen, Y.C., Myhre, G.B.: Chemical burns to the eye. Tidsskr Nor Laegeforen **124**(1), 49–51 (2004)
23. http://acto.de/media/pdf/EVEIT-%20ISOT%20 2006-zusammenfassung.swf
24. Kompa, S., Schareck, B., Tympner, J., Wustemeyer, H., Schrage, N.F.: Comparison of emergency eye-wash products in burned porcine eyes. Graefes Arch Clin Exp Ophthalmol **240**(4), 308–313 (2002)
25. Rihawi, S., Frentz, M., Schrage, N.F.: Emergency treatment of eye burns: which rinsing solution should we choose? Graefes Arch Clin Exp Ophthalmol **244**(7), 845–854 (2006)
26. Cejkova, J., Stipek, S., Crkovska, J., Ardan, T.: Changes of superoxide dismutase, catalase and glutathione peroxidase in the corneal epithelium after UVB rays. Histochemical and biochemical study. Histol Histopathol **15**(4), 1043–1050 (2000)
27. Hermel, M., Heckelen, A., Kirchhof, B., Schrage, N.F.: Inhibitory effect of ascorbic acid on human retinal pigment epithelial cell proliferation compared to cytostatic drugs–influence of histamine. Inflamm Res **50**(Suppl 2), S93–S95 (2001)
28. Maurer, J.K., Molai, A., Parker, R.D., Li, L., Carr, G.J., Petroll, W.M., Cavanagh, H.D., Jester, J.V.: Pathology of ocular irritation with bleaching agents in the rabbit low-volume eye test. Toxicol Pathol **29**(3), 308–319 (2001)
29. Yuen, H.K., Yeung, B.Y., Wong, T.H., Wu, W.K., Lam, D.S.: Descemet membrane detachment caused by hydrogen peroxide injury. Cornea **23**(4), 409–411 (2004)
30. Watt, B.E., Proudfoot, A.T., Vale, J.A.: Hydrogen peroxide poisoning. Toxicol Rev **23**(1), 51–57 (2004)
31. Beiran, I., Miller, B., Bentur, Y.: The efficacy of calcium gluconate in ocular hydrofluoric acid burns. Hum Exp Toxicol **16**(4)), 223–228 (1997)
32. Hojer, J., Personne, M., Hulten, P., Ludwigs, U.: Topical treatments for hydrofluoric acid burns: a blind controlled experimental study. J Toxicol Clin Toxicol **40**(7), 861–866 (2002)
33. Mathieu, L., Nehles, J., Blomet, J., Hall, A.H.: Efficacy of hexafluorine for emergent decontamination of hydrofluoric acid eye and skin splashes. Vet Hum Toxicol **43**(5), 263–265 (2001)
34. Söderberg, K., Kuusinen, P., Mathieu, L., Hall, A.H.: Hexafluorine®: An improved method for emergency decontamination of ocular and dermal hydrofluoric acid splashes. Vet Hum Toxicol **46**(4), 216–218 (2004)
35. Hall, A.H., Blomet, J., Gross, M., Nehles, J.: Hexafluorine® for emergency decontamination of hydrofluoric acid eye/skin splashes. Semiconductor Safety Assoc J **14**, 30–33 (2000)
36. Spöler, F., Frentz, M., Först, M., Kurz, H., Schrage, N.F.: Analysis of hydrofluoric acid penetration and decontamination of the eye by means of time-resolved optical coherence tomography. Burns **34**(4), 549–555 (2008). Epub 2007 Sep 14
37. Wilson, G.: Effect of hydrogen peroxide on epithelial light-scattering and stromal deturgescence. CLAO J **16**(1), S11–S14 (1990). discussion S14–S15
38. Luo, L., Li, D.Q., Corrales, R.M., Pflugfelder, S.C.: Hyperosmolar saline is a proinflammatory stress on the mouse ocular surface. Eye Contact Lens **31**(5), 186 (2005)
39. Lee, S.J., Jang, J.W., Lee, W.C., Kim, D.W., Jun, J.B., Bae, H.I., Kim, D.J.: Perforating disorder caused by salt-water application and its experimental induction. Int J Dermatol **44**(3), 210–214 (2005)
40. Langefeld, S., Reim, M., Redbrake, C., Schrage, N.F.: The corneal stroma: an inhomogeneous structure. Graefes Arch Clin Exp Ophthalmol **235**(8), 480–485 (1997)
41. http://www.acto.de – Verätzungen, download
42. Rihawi, S., Frentz, M., Schrage, N.F.: Emergency treatment of eye burns: which rinsing solution should we choose? Graefes Arch Clin Exp Ophthalmol **20**, 1–10 (2005)
43. Rihawi, S., Schrage, N., Frentz, M.: (ARVO Poster)
44. Pospisil, H., Holzhuetter, H.G.: A compartment Model to calculate time-dependent concentration profiles of topically applied chemical compounds in the a nteriro compartments of the rabbit eye. ATLA **29**, 347–365 (2001)
45. Reim, M.: Ein neues Behandlungskonzept für schwere Verätzungen. Klin Monatsbl Augenheilk vol. 196, n°1, pp. 1–5 (1990)
46. Tseng, S.C., Prabhasawat, P., Barton, K., Gray, T., Meller, D.: Amniotic membrane transplantation with or without limbal allografts for corneal surface reconstruction in patients with limbal stem cell deficiency. Arch Ophthalmol **116**(4), 431–441 (1998)
47. Pirouzmanesh, A., Herretes, S.P., Suwan-Apichon, O., Reyes, J.M.G., Cano, M., Gehlbach, P., Duh, E., Gurewitsch, E., Behrens, A.: Use of topical human amniotic fluid in the treatment of acute alkali burns of the eye ooster. ARVO Abstracts No 2722 Fort Lauderdale ARVO meeting 2006.
48. Sikder, S., Herretes, S.P., Gehlbach, P., Gurewitsch, E., Behrens, A.: Topical human amniotic: inhibition of induced corneal neovascularization. ARVO Abstracts No 1650 Fort Lauderdale ARVO meeting 2006.
49. Wilbanks, G.A., Streilein, J.W.: Fluids from immune privileged sites endow macrophages with the capacity to induce antigen-specific immune deviation via a mechanism involving transforming growth factor-beta. Eur J Immunol **22**(4), 1031–1036 (1992)
50. Reim, M., Kottek, A.A., Schrage, N.F.: The cornea surface and wound healing. Prog Retin Eye Res **16**(2), 183–225 (1997)
51. Chung, J.H.: Healing of rabbit corneal alkali wounds in vitro. Cornea **9**(1), 36–40 (1990)

52. Reim, M., Bahrke, C., Kuckelkorn, R., Kuwert, T.: Investigation of enzyme activities in severe burns of the anterior eye segment. Graefes Arch Clin Exp Ophthalmol **231**(5), 308–312 (1993)
53. Becker, J., Salla, S., Dohmen, U., Redbrake, C., Reim, M.: Explorative study of interleukin levels in the human cornea. Graefes Arch Clin Exp Ophthalmol **233**(12), 766–771 (1995)
54. Invest Ophthalmol Vis Sci. 2004 Nov; 45(11):3964-73
55. Ventura, A.C., Bohnke, M.: Pentoxifylline influences the autocrine function of organ cultured donor corneas and enhances endothelial cell survival. Br J Ophthalmol **85**(9), 1110–1114 (2001)
56. Paysse, E.A., Hamill, M.B., Koch, D.D., Hussein, M.A., Brady McCreery, K.M., Coats, D.K.: Epithelial healing and ocular discomfort after photorefractive keratectomy in children. J Cataract Refract Surg **29**(3), 478–481 (2003)
57. Reim, M.: The results of ischemia in chemical injuries. Eye **6**(4), 376–380 (1992)
58. Den, S., Sotozono, C., Kinoshita, S., Ikeda, T.: Efficacy of early systemic betamethasone or cyclosporin A after corneal alkali injury via inflammatory cytokine reduction. Acta Ophthalmol Scand **82**(2), 195–199 (2004)
59. Yamada, J., Dana, M.R., Sotozono, C., Kinoshita, S.: Local suppression of IL-1 by receptor antagonist in the rat model of corneal alkali injury. Exp Eye Res **76**(2), 161–167 (2003)

Rinsing Therapy of Eye Burns

Norbert Schrage

Rinsing is the most outstanding early measure to set up in order to prevent further propagation of the corrosive to the eye and to remove the later on disaster-producing inflammatory proteins and mediators in the clinical course of treatments with a lower frequency. This is a well-known and trained fact in all official recommendations all over the world concerning first aid in eye burns (ANSI Standards and Recommendations of the Berufsgenossenschaften in Germany). Cleaning with any watery fluid of pH below 9 and over 5, with temperature limits between 10 to 42°C, seems in first line to be acceptable if no other specified fluids are available. The most outstanding treatment factor, except from the fluid, is the time of intervention [1]. If early treatment is done within the first seconds, the decontamination can be completed before the immersion of the tissue, and the disaster of severe burns requires real intratissular decontamination strategies [2] to prevent intraocular burns [3]. There are basic considerations on type, action, and composition of fluids that are demonstrated in the following subchapters.

This was not a subject of systematic research except the approval that phosphate buffer was preferred due to data of the 1970s from Laux [4]. Up to now, there is only one scientific prove out of chemical neutralization experiments on borate buffer, phosphate buffer, or Diphoterine® in the beaker [5]. In clinical context, there is only one systematic study of Merle and Gerard who performed a prospective study comparing saline solution and rinsing with Diphoterine® in a clinical trial [6].

6.1 Important

To have a precise scientific insight into the action of rinsing fluids, we have to be aware of the mechanisms involved, which are:

- Dilution
- Diffusion
- Chemical reaction
- Osmolar regulation of the tissues
- Remnants from any chemical process

To elucidate this, for example, the eye burn with 2M sodium hydroxide is known to change osmolarity (1,800 mOsmol/kg) and propagates by diffusion into the tissue (See OCT images at Sect. 5.1.6 and Fig. 5.12). Spreading into the tissue results in immediate saponification of the cellular membranes and lysis of collagen to gelatin and low molecular breakdown products that have been identified by Pfister to be the origin of proinflammatory responses [7]. Furthermore, we have shown in the experimental part of Chap. 5 (See Sect. 5.2.6 and Figs. 5.16 and 5.17) that the release of mediators is the origin of the additional biological response.

To have insight into these mechanisms, we have performed and published several experiments on diffusion of corrosive, rinsing with different osmolar solutions to check the influence of osmolar conditioning of the cornea [8]. Further, we have tried to evaluate the diffusion of corrosive throughout the cornea [9]. In the latest experiments being published under www.acto.de, we present the effect of fluids of different osmolarities and their action on cells. Unpublished data give insight into

N. Schrage
Head of the Department Professorship at the RWTH Aachen, Founder of ACTO (Aachen Center of Technology Transfer in Ophthalmology), Department of Ophthalmology of the City Hospital, Augenklinik Köln Merheim, Cologne, Germany
e-mail: schrage@acto.de

the cellular resistance to pH changes in iso-osmolar tissue culture media. We worked out a systematic series of measurements of the pH neutralizing action of any type of rinsing fluid available in the market. These series included tap water, saline, borate, phosphate in different formulations, and Diphoterine®.

6.2 Mechanisms of Diffusion in Rinsing Therapy

If any corrosive touches the corneal surface, it first breaks into the tear fluid film; later, the tight junctions of the epithelium have to be broken after the epithelium is denuded from the surface. The propagation through the corneal stroma is limited by the architecture of homogenous lamellae. To classify the speed and variation of propagation into the cornea, special measurements are required. These measurements rely on the first change of pH of the aqueous humor which is close to the endothelium. They are made with a pH electrode. By these measurements, in eye burns with 50 µL of 2M NaOH, we have found a relatively stable speed of diffusion through the corneal stroma of 5–8 µm/s. By this, the time of damage of the endothelium starting with a severe rising of pH can be confirmed to be around 80–100 s from the initial eye burn of the corneal surface. The propagation of the corrosive with intraocular pH change follows a stable pattern with a consecutive severe pH change throughout all layers of the cornea. The work of Pospisil et al. [10] opens a theoretical model that explains the introduction of corrosives into the eye and the outflow of these materials by the diffusion. The model still lacks the influence of distribution coefficient changes due to the alteration by severe corrosives and the influence of other substances introducing chemical interaction like neutralization, amphoteric binding, or precipitation of unsoluble salts. We can observe by high-resolution real time optical coherence tomography (OCT) the diffusion of hydrofluoric acid into the cornea (Fig. 6.1). The mechanistic understanding of the inflow is relatively completed, but the decontamination is still not understood by means of mathematical models. This necessitates more work in the near future.

6.3 Osmolar Effects in Rinsing Therapy

The effects of osmolarity on cells are well known from physiology. Semipermeable membranes allow a water flux depending on the number of solved ions. Therefore, a cell with its own tissue osmolarity of about

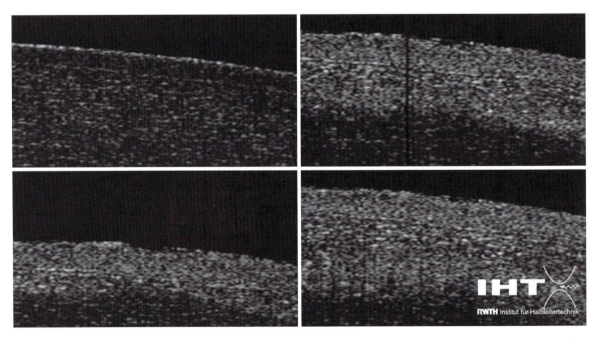

Fig. 6.1 HF diffusion within the cornea during an observation time of 30 min reaching the corneal endothelium (micrographs done by the IHT group of Prof. Dr. Kurz and Dipl. Ing. Spöler)

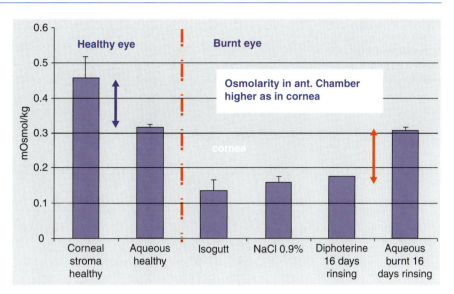

Fig. 6.2 Healthy corneal stroma, aqueous fluid, and corneal stroma osmolarities after prolonged 16 day treatment with phosphate buffer (Isogutt®), saline solution, and Diphoterine®

420 mOsmol/kg in the cornea [11] will swell if tap water is applied to a denuded stroma, where epithelial tight junctions normally prevent water influx [12]. This is the deeper origin of well-known surgical corneal swelling due to hypoosmolar rinsing fluids in damaged epithelial cells. Here lies the origin of Descemets folds and corneal clouding directly after eye burns and water flushing [13]. The osmolarity of highly dissociated corrosives is directly dependent on their molarity and dissociation constants. Exceeding concentrations of dissociating fluids of more than 420 mOsmol/kg will result in a water loss directly due to the trauma and a consecutive severe edema after flushing with hypoosmolar water [8]. For cellular populations loaded with ions over their normal levels, there is a considerable evidence that low osmolarity will destroy cell borders.

There are several most interesting observations concerning osmolarity. We have found that there is an important difference of osmolarity between the hyperosmolar stroma with 420 mOsmol/kg and the extra and intraocular fluids with lower osmolarities of about 320 mOsmol/kg. This results in an inversion of the water flux, when barriers like endothelium and epithelium are damaged. The immediate result of any membrane damage is that water starts to flow from the outside into the corneal stroma. This results in a corneal edema with turbidity. This is an indirect proof of the pumping function of the endothelium.

In several experiments, we have measured the corneal stroma and intracameral osmolarity by means of cryo milling and redilution of the stroma of the burnt cornea and by direct measurements of the intraocular fluids.

We have observed the following pattern (Fig. 6.2) of decrease of the tissue osmolarity after eye burns within the corneal stroma. This confirms the clinical finding of severe edema of the stroma and was sustained by work of Kompa et al. [8], who have found the alteration of the corneal swelling and corneal osmolarity by the eye burn itself and changes due to different fluids used for rinsing of the cornea thereafter.

All burnt corneal stroma show lower osmolarity due to the loss of ions by continuous rinsing. The higher osmolar Diphoterine® adds some ions to the burnt corneal stroma, but its osmolarity is still much lower than the one of the aqueous humor. It is obvious that there is no change in osmolarity in aqeous humor in healthy and in burnt eyes due to autoregulation of this milieu by the ciliary body secretion. The considerable differences in tissue osmolarity indicate that there will be a strong fluid uptake into the corneal tissue, resluting in opacity. This indicates a severe water uptake and a lack of the endothelial pumping function.

This severe water uptake is confirmed by the next figure (Fig. 6.3) showing the hydration of the cornea after burn that is kept untreated for up to 7 days or respectively treated by three times daily rinsing of the eye with phosphate buffer (Isogutt®), saline solution, or Diphoterine® solution for 16 days.

The untreated eye burns result in a severe and high water uptake. With rinsing therapy, this does not really change to a large extent after 16 days. The lower hydration in the phosphate group is due to the calcification and loss of stromal ground substance that is able to swell.

Fig. 6.3 Water contents of healthy and burnt cornea. The hydration level is obtained as follows: (dry mass (g) + water (g))/ water (g)

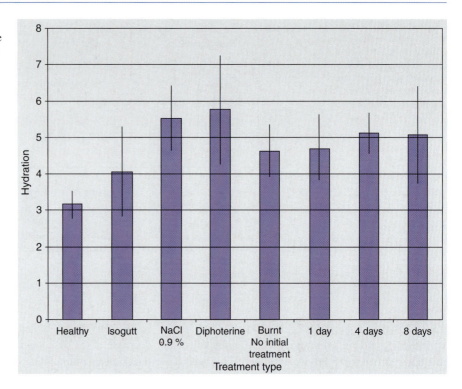

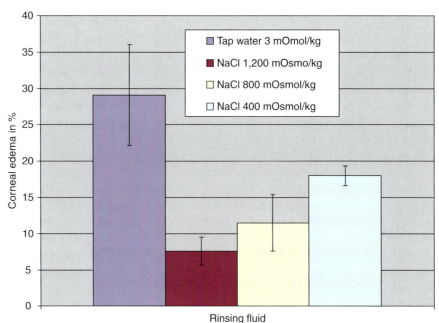

Fig. 6.4 Osmolarity of different rinsing solutions

The reversal of the osmolarity-caused corneal swelling after eye burns is not possible by increasing osmolarities in the rinsing fluids as tried with saline solutions with different osmolarities (Fig. 6.4). The result of this experiment is that, even with the highest osmolarities, the reversal of the stromal edema is not completely possible, but a higher amount of initial swelling can be prevented. Even with 1,200 mOsmol/kg rinsing, the thickness of the burnt cornea increases by 5%, thus showing the uptake of water.

Osmolar effects lead to cell lysis as we can demonstrate in epithelial (ARPE19) and mesenchymal

6.3 Osmolar Effects in Rinsing Therapy

cell (murine fibroblasts L929) cultures, thereby, in rinsing of cellular tissues that are immersed with 800 mOsmol/kg, which is twice as much the normal 360–420 mOsmol/kg in cell culture medium.

It has been found that the osmolar stress releases Interleukins from cells and has an intrinsic proinflammatory action.

The cell lysis that we observed in rinsing experiments liberates fragments of cells and necrotic material leading to fast inflammation.

In Fig. 6.5, tissue culture preincubated with 800 mOsmol (NaCl), shows cells of normal shape and function.

The same tissue culture after exposure to tap water, with blown-up cells after 60 s of water exposure is shown in Fig. 6.6.

After 120 s of exposure, it is shown with total cytolysis and necrosis (Fig. 6.7).

If any rinsing solution that is isotonic to blood such as 0.9% NaCl or RINGER lactate is applied, the result of cellular damage will be different. The cells blow up but keep their integrity.

Tissue culture incubated with RINGER lactate of 290 mOsmol is shown in Fig.6.8. Cells are blown up, but still, membranes are of good integrity (Fig. 6.8).

Higher osmolarities in early rinsing have effect on the integrity of cells and stabilize the cellular bodies against the water influx. This concept is realized by Diphoterine® of 820 mOsmol.

Tissue culture is preincubated with 800 mOsmol (NaCl) and contains cells of normal shape and function.

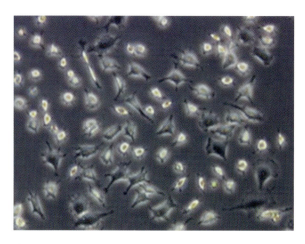

Fig. 6.5 Tissue culture preincubated with 800 mOsmol (NaCl)

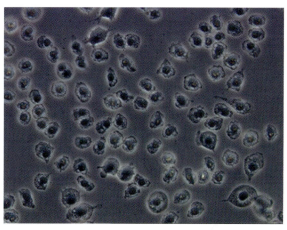

Fig. 6.7 After 120 s of exposure with total cytolysis and necrosis

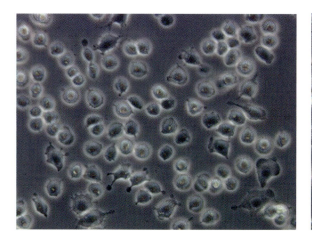

Fig. 6.6 The same tissue culture after exposure to tap water

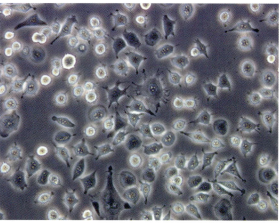

Fig. 6.8 The cells blow up

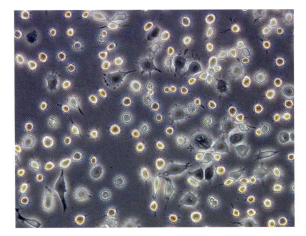

Fig. 6.9 Tissue culture preincubated with Diphoterine®

The same tissue culture is incubated with Diphoterine® of 820 mOsmol (Fig. 6.9), and shows cells with a stabilized low volume and without any lack of integrity.

On the other hand, the observations made by Kompa et al. in tissue swelling dependency after eye burns give insight into the reality after burns. We have rinsed corneas of homogenous burns with different osmolar solutions from 0 to 1,200 mOsmol NaCl; further, we have tried to use the standard corneal deswelling media to cure direct postburn edema. None of the substances could return the normal corneal thickness. This indicates that the swelling is only one part of the real damage. The structural changes lead to a water uptake and a change in the distribution of the intra-extracellular water compartment. Furthermore, the swelling of the cornea was directly correlated to the osmolarity of the rinsing solution. The most outstanding swelling was produced by tap water, the least one by a 1,200 mOsmol NaCl solution. There was a direct correlation between the corneal osmolarity at the end of rinsing and the solution's osmolarity. Therefore, we dare to speak of "ional conditioning" of the cornea after eye burns. Other solutions that are used for rinsing, such as mannitol, condensed serum of high osmolarity, milk, and others, have behaved in the same manner as mentioned above. The deswelling function must be considered of highest interest due to the fact that the corneal swelling seems to be a decisive factor on later corneal scars [14]. From that point of view, preventing corneal swelling soon after the first rinsing is the most important measure.

6.3.1 Types of Irrigation Fluids

There are different types of irrigation fluids. We distinguish between water, ion-containing nonbuffering and buffering solutions, and amphoteric solutions. All water-containing solutions are able to decontaminate by dilution and washing of any surface. If using an ion-containing solution, the osmolarity increases and swelling decreases. This results in assuming stable diffusion processes, that is, with increase of the thickness of a burnt cornea by water rinsing, the arrival of the corrosive into the endothelium is delayed and vice versa. With high ionic contents the time of the first rise in the anterior chamber is earlier. These theoretical evaluations are confirmed in practical experiments done and published by Rihawi et al. [5]. Moreover, there is another aspect, mentioned in ophthalmologic literature, that solutions exceeding an osmolarity of 600 cause pain to the eye [15]. This is due to free nerve endings within the cornea that especially react to osmolar stress. We have tried to evaluate this phenomenon with the hyperosmolar Diphoterine® that was used to rinse healthy eyes (ethic committee commitment) and have found that there is no evidence for this special fluid to cause pain.

A well-known fact to plunge into a sweat water basin after high osmolar stress, itching and burning after first reopening of the eyes. This is well explainable by means of the severe osmolar shock of tissues and surviving nerve endings if such measures are taken.

6.4 Effect of Irrigation Fluids

The overall effect of irrigation fluids can be measured by their respective capacity to decontaminate the eye surface and to increase the time lapse of intervention. Moreover the most important is that the rinsing fluid must save vision and prevent secondary disease after eye burns. How to reach this?

First of all, we have to consider the electrolytic contents of the commercially available solutions which are compared in the following diagram (Fig. 6.10).

We try to compare the existing solutions in the market based on their capacities of treating eye burns to know which solution improves the time to treatment. We used a standardized model of eye burns and

6.4 Effect of Irrigation Fluids

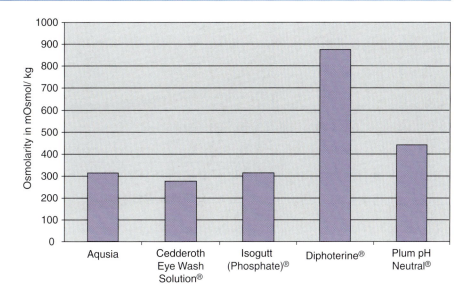

Fig. 6.10 Osmolarities of commercially available eye rinsing solutions

following decontamination. Eye burns was routinely done with 50 μL of 2M NaOH placed in a soaked 10 mm diameter filter paper on the cornea for 20 s. The anterior chamber was canulated with a micro pH electrode and the movement of the anterior chamber pH was continuously monitored. With this approach, we could prove that there is a dependency of pH change in the anterior chamber, with a slower rise of the anterior chamber pH when rinsed with water. This first minute advantage is followed by a fixed and high intraocular pH for a long time. With Ringer lactate, saline solution, and phosphate buffer, the situation is even worse, because there is an initial fast rise of intraocular pH and no return to normal. The situation is completely different for borate buffer (Cederoths Eye Wash solution®), which is less effective on bases and Diphoterine® solution, which is as effective on acids as it is on bases. After a fast initial rise of the intracameral pH, it drops and is returned to about 9.5 at the end of a 15 min rinsing period. It is the same for corneal calcifying products, only mentioned here for completeness and not for recommendation, such as the phosphate buffer "pH neutral®" from Plum®.

As the cornea physiologically contains almost no phosphate, we have found evidence that for an osmolar conditioning of the cornea, an electrolyte conditioning is highly probable. We could prove this by means of Energy dispersive X-ray analysis (EDXA) [16]. With this method, we have found elevated phosphate contents in the cornea after rinsing one or several times with phosphate buffer [17]. This reflects a situation of introduction of foreign elements in the cornea that are known to cause side effects especially if the chemical reaction leads to precipitation of new and non-organotypic salts.

The comparison of all rinsing fluid based on their effect on the anterior chamber pH is presented in the following figures. All experiments were repeated five times and mean and standard deviation are given to elucidate the variance of the experimental set up. There is clear evidence that only some solutions buffer acids and alkali (Figs. 6.11–6.13). These solutions are polyvalent and are Diphoterine® and the phosphate buffer of higher concentration like the plum pH neutral. Borate buffer has a high capacity to buffer alkali but a low capacity to buffer acids.

The curves represent the intraocular pH over time measured on real rabbit eyes that are burnt with 50 μL of 2M NaOH for 20 min and on the cornea for 20 s with a filter paper. The rinsing solutions were applied for 15 min with a flow of 66 mL/min. All curves represent five repeated experiments. Original data were published by Rihawi et al. in 2005. There is a considerable later onset of pH rise with low osmolarity rinsing and a lower extent of pH rise with tap water rinsing and an earlier onset of pH rise in all solutions containing ions like saline, Diphoterine®, phosphate buffer, and RINGER lactate.

We have found that all the active solutions have a good action on the intraocular pH, but all the solutions containing electrolytes considerably increase the initial intraocular pH. Therefore, from the point of

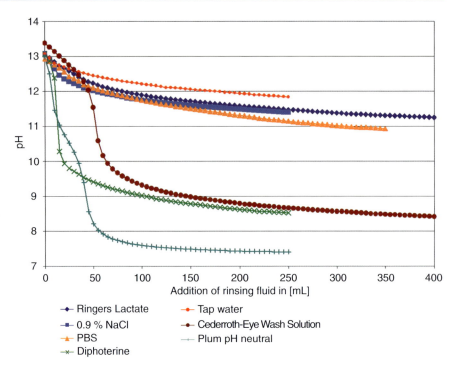

Fig. 6.11 Buffer capacity on alkali of the commercially available rinsing fluids

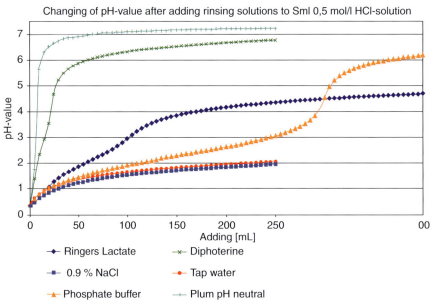

Fig. 6.12 Buffer capacity on acids of the commercially available rinsing fluids

osmolar stabilization of cells, osmolar stabilization is desired but low initial osmolarities with water tend to have lower peaks of initial pH. To prevent shock, like changes of osmolarity, we propose stabilizing cells with osmolar proteinic or sugar components to prevent electrolytes to promote invasion of corrosives and to treat the cornea better.

The overall question on improving treatment is not yet answered. Up to now, there is little knowledge on corrosive type, extent and time of exposure of tissues ans cells which could be acceptable. In the same order, there is up to now no description on how and when a treatment is predictable as successful and when it will not prevent damage.

6.4 Effect of Irrigation Fluids

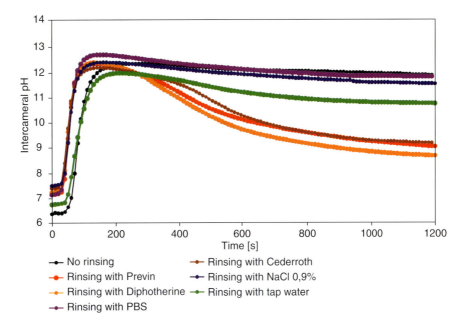

Fig. 6.13 Intracameral pH after corneal rinsing with the commercially available rinsing fluids

To evaluate these questions that are on one hand related to the corrosive and on the other hand related to the biological and chemical response to an accidental exposure, we have tried to set up experiments to give insight into the questions.

First, we have tried to evaluate the resistance of cells toward pH changes without a change of osmolarity. This major precaution has to be taken, because, otherwise, the results would have been changed by two different parameters.

In a setup of cell culture, we have found that tissue culture medium salts (Earls salts) can be replaced by NaOH or HCl and water within a range of pH 2–11.3 without changing the 350 mOsmol/kg osmolarity of the medium. Therefore, the experimental setup does not interfere by means of semipermeable membranes with the water content of the cells.

We have exposed non-confluent cell cultures with 50,000 cells/mL attached to the cell culture bottle and introduced a medium exchange for 1 h. The medium was exchanged with pH from 2, 3, 4, 5 and 9, 10, 11, 11.3. We have observed acute changes and after a period of 1 h, the pH-conditioned medium was withdrawn and replaced by a tissue culture medium. The overall conclusion of these experiments show that pH must be returned to less than 9 and higher than 5 within less than 60 min and preferably within 30 min. This is achieved by the results are given in Fig. 6.14.

L929 cells were exposed to osmolar stable solutions with variation of pH from 11.3 to 9.5 for 64 min. After this time, the medium was changed to normal MEM and the surviving cells were counted 24 h later. For pH over 10.75, a significant loss of cells can be detected after 1 h; 24 h later, no regrowth occurs on these cells.

The interpretation of these experiments is that the cellular growth in unconditioned medium results in the proliferation of cells after 24 h. The same result can be seen for cells incubated at pH 10, 10.5, and 10.75. Only pH 9 results in a lower proliferation rate indicating a slow growth. Therefore, we believe that the exposure to higher pHs results in an inadequate proliferation that should be prevented.

L929 cells were exposed to osmolar stable solutions with variation of pH from 5 to 2 for 64 min. After this time, the medium was changed to normal MEM and the surviving cells were counted 24 h later (Fig. 6.15).

For pH below 5, no visible significant loss of cells can be detected after 1 h, but only some cells have survived after an exposition to pH above 5 after 24 h. We conclude that a pH below 5 must be regarded as mostly critical for more than 60 min of exposure.

The difference between acidic and alkaline exposure for cell cultures is striking. The reproliferation after 24 h is completely missing in all groups below 5, whereas cells exposed to pH above 9 and below 11 tend to show a good proliferation. This indicates that a strong decrease

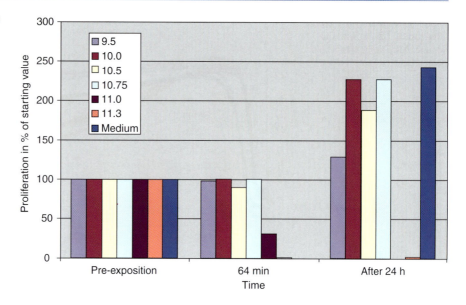

Fig. 6.14 Exposure of L929 cells to osmolar stable solutions with variation of pH from 11.3 to 9.5 for 64 min

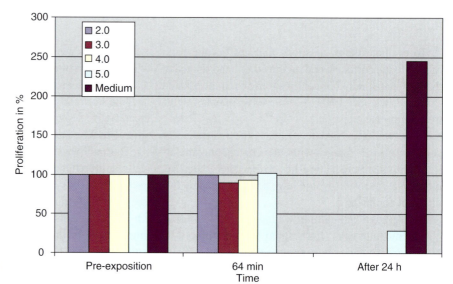

Fig. 6.15 Exposure of L929 cells to osmolar stable solutions with variation of pH from 5 to 2 for 64 min

of the pH in the anterior chamber of the eye is much more harmful than the elevation above 9.

6.5 High End Decontamination

6.5.1 Peroxides and Radicals Decontamination

We have found in some preliminary experiments that the decontamination of peroxides is insufficient with buffers, due to missing action on these substrates. Therefore, we have examined drugs known for peroxide decontamination such as Dimercaprol, Vitamin C, and Tocopherol. Similar experiments were made with Diphoterine®. Our investigation aims to the restoration of the glutathione equilibrium in the exposed corneal tissue without any regeneration capacity of the tissue itself. These experiments were performed on homogenates of porcine corneas that were exposed to hydrogen peroxide and nitric acid and then treated with the different drugs. The results, given in Fig. 6.16, show a clear restoration when using Diphoterine®.

The measurements of glutathione reflect the total capacity of decontamination of oxidative stress within the cornea. The glutathione system gives the outer

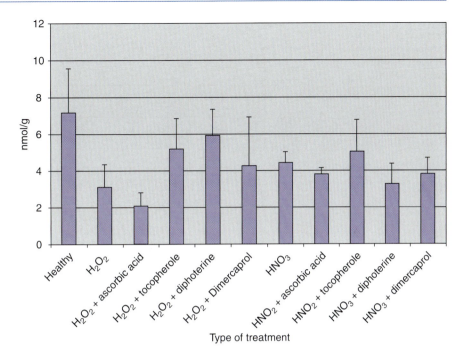

Fig. 6.16 Glutathione content after treatment of corneal homogenates with hydrogen peroxide or HNO_3

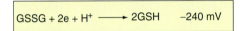

Fig. 6.17 The glutathione system

limits of oxidation and reduction by supplying the glutathione peroxidase with a redox potential [18] (Fig. 6.17).

All decontaminations of radicals within the body are operated by means of structural changes of ascorbate, β-carotin, or tocopherol. Those reactive partners known as the antioxidative system are all regenerated by the glutathione system. Therefore, this system gives a good overview on the oxidative state of a tissue (Fig. 6.18).

The reversal of the glutathione is not achieved by all substances and a considerable loss is produced by the agents.

The ratio of glutathione to reduced glutathione is reestablished only by Dimercaprol and Diphoterine® (Fig. 6.19).

The above-presented charts give a clear indication that none of the commercially available drugs or medical devices is able to protect the cornea from changes due to strong reducing agents or oxidants. Except this, the restoration of an equilibrium of reduced glutathione (GSH) and oxidized glutathione (GSSG) provides source of peroxidic decontamination for the tissue.

Thus with Diphoterine® and Dimercaprol, there is a considerable improvement of the physiological capacity of chemical decontamination. By this, the use of polyvalent solutions in first aid offers a considerable advantage as the best currently available treatments.

With the concept of Diphoterine®, even the restoration of glutathione contents in the burnt cornea can be achieved without any action of the regenerating tissues. This is a major value. Dimercaprol has similar effects and might be an opportune alternative, but this drug does not act on alkali and acids as well as the buffers and amphoteric substances do.

6.5.2 Hydrofluoric Acid Decontamination

In recent work, we could give proof of different decontamination strategies from conventional water rinsing over calcium gluconate to the rinsing with the specific fluoride decontaminating rinsing solution Hexafluorine®. The specific complexation due to HF action on tissue results in the total loss of calcium within seconds as shown in cell cultures in Chap. 5 (Sect. 5.1.4, Fig. 5.9a and b). By means of photography in the ex vivo eye irritation assay and by means of Optical coherence tomography, we could give clear indication of the efficiency of the decontamination with Hexafluorine® (Fig. 6.20).

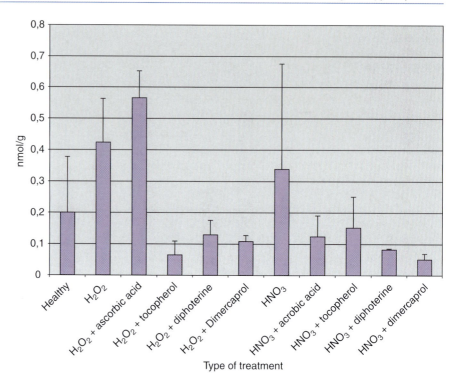

Fig. 6.18 Glutathione reduced content after treatment of corneal homogenate with hydrogen peroxide or HNO_3

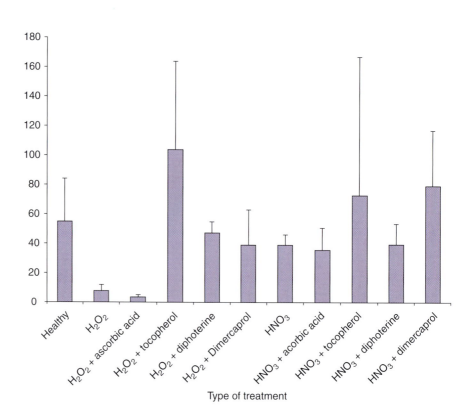

Fig. 6.19 Ratio of glutathione/reduced glutathione

6.5 High End Decontamination

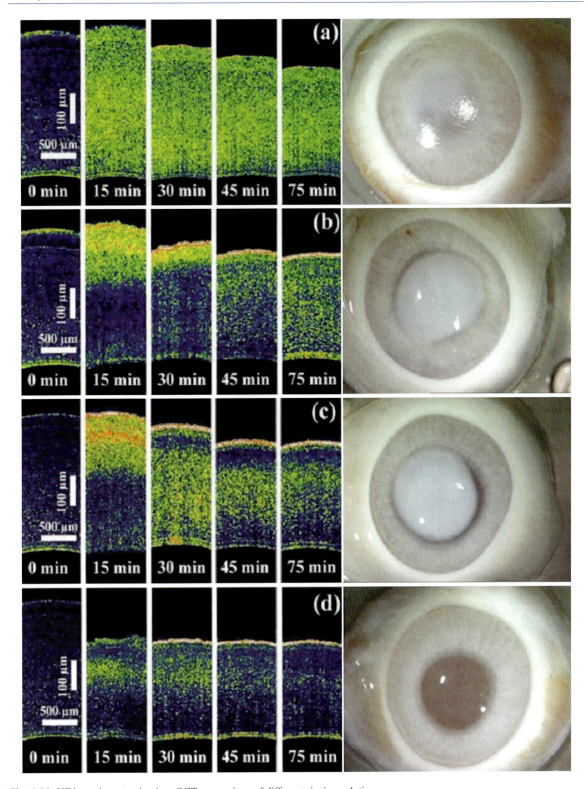

Fig. 6.20 HF burn decontamination: OCT comparison of different rinsing solutions

Rinsing of 20 s, 25 μL, 2.5% HF burns with different fluids: (a) no rinsing, (b) rinsing with tap water for 15 min, (c) rinsing with calcium gluconate 2% for 15 min, and (d) rinsing with Anti HF solution (Hexafluorine®) for 15 min.

It is obvious that the corneal opacity from HF-Ca complexes is completely absent in the case of rinsing with Hexafluorine® solution. There is a clear corneal opacity in all other rinsing solutions (a–c) [19].

6.6 Side Effects of Rinsing Solutions in the Treatment of Eye Burns

We know from basic data that the cornea does not contain many elements except Na, Cl, S, lower contents of Ca, Mg, and P mostly in the epithelial layer. These data have been published by our group (Langefeld et al.). By introducing corrosives onto the cornea, the corneal elemental constitution is severely altered by means of introducing high concentrations of the corrosive. This has been exemplarily shown by von Fischern et al. [17]. Mostly, the corneal water content and the corneal electrolyte constitution change after eye burns. This is even more the case if rinsing solutions used in the therapy introduce elements or substances that precipitate into the cornea, as shown for phosphate buffer in dry eyes [20] and later on by our group for phosphate buffer application on burnt eyes [21, 22]. The same situation occurs with HF with precipitates of $CaCl_2$ in case of Calcium gluconate application. The problem of precipitates in the cornea is the in-transparency and the long-term deposition of such infiltrates hindering optical rehabilitation.

Latest results on secondary effects of rinsing solutions containing phosphate buffer in treating eye burns [21] were confirmed by studies of dry eye treatment with phosphate-containing eye drops published by Bernauer et al. [20].

Therefore, we recommend phosphate-free solutions for any therapy on the eye including rinsing. Other elements like Borate within the Cederoth Eye Wash® solution or citrate like used by Pfister do not precipitate with the known chemical corrosives. Therefore, these elements are considered as uncritical due to the later diffusion-mediated disappearance of the rinsing fluids as described by the Pospisil model [10]. Figures 6.21 and 6.22 show the effect of a single

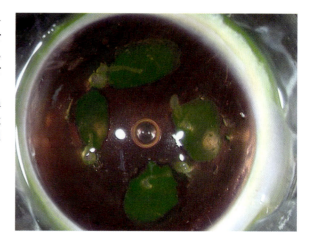

Fig. 6.21 Scratched cornea

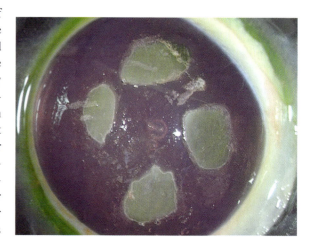

Fig. 6.22 Corneal calcifications

rinsing with Plum pH neutral on an ex vivo cornea that has been cultivated for more than 2 days after the initial erosion and rinsing for 15 min. The local surface treatment was one drop artificial tears every hour for 2 days. A clear corneal superficial calcification is visible.

Secondary effects of irrigation fluids: ex vivo eye irritation assay with four scratches on the cornea, incubated for 2 days and treated with artificial tears containing $CaCl_2$ in 0.13 mmol/L concentration each 24 drops per day with 30 min of interval between phosphate and tear application. Second image is taken after 2 days with obvious corneal calcification.

Similar calcifications were seen after eye burns and treatment with Isogutt® eye rinsing solution for 48 h continued as recommended by Laux [4]. We have found this case and earlier reported it on systematic review in these cases [22]. These *ex vivo* and clinical results were endorsed by an experimental work done by our group on rabbits being rinsed several times with phosphate buffer [23].

6.7 Our Expectations

There are three major issues that should be addressed in the near future:

The decontamination and healing after burns must be subjected to systematic research. Thus we have started with healing in the ex vivo eye irritation assay EVEIT® after mechanical and chemical exposures. The healing is monitored by biochemistry and optical coherence tomography.

The inflammatory reaction around eye burns has been subject of older research and might be more elucidated by means of modern technologies of microassays on molecular and proteinic levels.

Last, the surgical procedures such as keratoprosthesis [24] surgery and corneal and limbal transplantations are on the way to be developed. Yet, the transfer of cultured stem cells is a problem due to the need of mouse-derived feeder cells; these might introduce new risks of disease transfer. Until those problems are not solved, these techniques are not applicable on humans, but these problems are likely to be solved in the near future [25].

The evaluation of chemical hazard and chemical action by means of the REACH activities in the European Union might be a useful source of future prospective evaluation of the probable eye burns due to chemicals.

References

1. Kuckelkorn, R., Kottek, A., Schrage, N., Reim, M.: Poor prognosis of severe chemical and thermal eye burns: the need for adequate emergency care and primary prevention. Int Arch Occup Environ Health **67**(4), 281–284 (1995)
2. Merle, H., Donnio, A., Ayeboua, L., Michel, F., Thomas, F., Ketterle, J., Leonard, C., Josset, P., Gerard, M.: Alkali ocular burns in Martinique (French West Indies) Evaluation of the use of an amphoteric solution as the rinsing product. Burns **31**(2), 205–211 (2005)
3. Kuckelkorn, R., Kottek, A., Reim, M.: Intraocular complications after severe chemical burns-incidence and surgical treatment. Klin Monatsbl Augenheilkd **205**(2), 86–92 (1994)
4. Laux, U., Roth, H.W., Krey, H., Steinhardt, B.: Die Wasserstoffkonzentration des Kammerwassers nach Alkaliverätzungen der Hornhaut und deren therapeutische Beeinflußbarkeit. Eine tierexperimentelle Studie. Albrecht von Graefes Arch Clin Exp Ophthalmol **195**(1), 33–40 (1975)
5. Rihawi, S., Frentz, M., Schrage, N.F.: Emergency treatment of eye burns: which rinsing solution should we choose? Graefes Arch Clin Exp Ophthalmol **244**(7), 845–854 (2006)
6. Gerard, M., Merle, H., Ayeboua, L., Richer, R.: Prospective study of eye burns at the Fort de France University Hospital. J Fr Ophtalmol **22**(8), 834–847 (1999). French
7. Pfister, R.R., Haddox, J.L., Sommers, C.I., Lam, K.W.: A neutrophil chemoattractant is released from cellular and extracellular components of the alkali-degraded cornea and blood. Invest Ophthalmol Vis Sci **37**(1), 230–237 (1996)
8. Kompa, S., Schareck, B., et al.: Comparison of emergency eye-wash products in burned porcine eyes. Graefes Arch Clin Exp Ophthalmol **240**(4), 308–313 (2002)
9. Schrage, N.F., Rihawi, R., Frentz, M., Reim, M.: Acute therapy for eye burns. Klin Monatsbl Augenheilkd. **221**(4), 253–261 (2004)
10. Pospisil, H., Holzhutter, H.G.: A compartment model to calculate time-dependent concentration profiles of topically applied chemical compounds in the anterior compartments of the rabbit eye. Altern Lab Anim **29**(3), 347–365 (2001)
11. Langefeld, S., Reim, M., Redbrake, C., Schrage, N.F.: The corneal stroma, an inhomogenous structure. Graefes Arch Clin Exp Ophthalmol **235**(8), 480–485 (1997)
12. Reim, M.: Surgical anatomy, physiology, biochemistry and questions on the inlay technique. Ophthalmologe **89**(2), 109–118 (1992)
13. Bramsen, T., Ehlers, N.: Early postoperative changes in graft thickness after penetrating keratoplasty. Influence of host corneal disorder on time course. Acta Ophthalmol (Copenh) **57**(2), 258–268 (1979)
14. Kubota, M., Fagerholm, P.: Corneal alkali burn in the rabbit. Waterbalance, healing and transparency. Acta Ophthalmol (Copenh) **69**(5), 635–640 (1991)
15. Reim, M. (ed.): Augenheilkunde, 5th edn. Enke, Stuttgart (1996)
16. Schrage, N.F., Benz, K., Beaujean, P., Burchard, W.G., Reim, M.: A simple empirical calibration of energy dispersive X-ray analysis (EDXA) on the cornea. Scanning Microsc **7**(3), 881–888 (1993)
17. von Fischern, T., Lorenz, U., Burchard, W.G., Reim, M., Schrage, N.F.: Changes in the mineral composition of the rabbit cornea after alkali burns. Graefes Arch Clin Exp Ophthalmol **236**(7), 553–558 (1998)
18. Aslund, F., Berndt, K.D., Holmgren, A.: Redox potentials of glutaredoxins and other thiol-disulfide oxidoreductases of the thioredoxin superfamily determined by direct protein-protein redox equilibria. J Biol Chem **272**(49), 30780–30786 (1997)
19. Spöler, F., Frentz, M., Först, M., Kurz, H., Schrage, N.F.: Analysis of hydrofluoric acid penetration and decontamination of the eye by means of time-resolved optical coherence tomography. Burns **34**(4), 549–555 (2008). doi:10.1016/j.burns.2007.05.004
20. Bernauer, W., Thiel, M.A., Kurrer, M., Heiligenhaus, A., Rentsch, K.M., Schmitt, A., Heinz, C., Yanar, A.: Corneal calcification following intensified treatment with sodium hyaluronate artificial tears. Br J Ophthalmol **90**(3), 285–288 (2006)

21. Kompa, S., Redbrake, C., Dunkel, B., Weber, A., Schrage, N.: Corneal calcification after chemical eye burns caused by eye drops containing phosphate buffer. Burns **32**(6), 744–747 (2006)
22. Schrage, N.F., Kompa, S., Ballmann, B., Reim, M., Langefeld, S.: Relationship of eye burns with calcifications of the cornea? Graefes Arch Clin Exp Ophthalmol **243**(8), 780–784 (2005)
23. Schrage, N.F., Schlossmacher, B., Aschenbernner, W., Langefeld, S.: Phosphate buffer in alkali eye burns as an inducer of experimental corneal calcification. Burns **27**(5), 459–464 (2001)
24. Kompa, S., Redbrake, C., Langefeld, S., Brenman, K., Schrage, N.: The type II Aachen-Keratoprosthesis in humans: case report of the first prolonged application. Int J Artif Organs **24**(2), 110–114 (2001)
25. Pellegrini, G., Traverso, C.E., Franzi, A.T., Zingirian, M., Cancedda, R., De Luca, M.: Long-term restoration of damaged corneal surfaces with autologous cultivated corneal epithelium. Lancet **349**(9057), 990–993 (1997)

The Clinical of Ocular Burns

Max Gérard

7.1 Few Reminders

As some readers with no special knowledge in ocular anatomy and physiology may read this chapter, it seems necessary to begin it with a few reminders.

7.1.1 Anatomy Reminder

Figures 7.1 and 7.2.[1]

The cornea and the bulbar conjunctiva together form the ocular surface, which is the group of tissues that is first damaged by chemical burns.

The cornea is the transparent window of the eye; it is 500 µm thick at the centre and histologically made of, from the surface to the inside:

- The corneal epithelium, constituted of five layers of cells, 20 µm thick, and forming the roof of the cornea
- The corneal stroma, made of collagen fibrillae interwoven according to a specific architecture (and between which are located some keratocytes), 450 µm thick; it is the framework of the
- The corneal endothelium constituted of one unique layer of cells, 5–10 µm thick

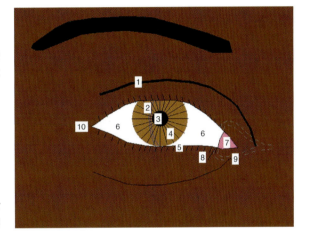

Fig. 7.1 Front view of the right eyeball. *1*, Upper eyelid crease; *2*, Cornea; *3*, Pupil; *4*, Iris; *5*, Lower eyelid margin; *6*, Bulbar conjunctiva; *7*, Lacrymal caruncle; *8*, Lacrymal meatus; *9*, Lacrymal caniculus; *10*, Lateral canthus

7.1.2 Physiology Reminder

The essential and specific property of the cornea is transparency. This transparency especially depends on:

- The quality of the lacrymal film.
- The histological architecture of the cornea and specifically that of the stroma.
- The evenness of the corneal surface.
- The absence of vascularization.

M. Gérard
Ophthalmologist, Medical director of Head
and Neck Unit, Department of Ophthalmology,
Cayenne Hospital, Cayenne, French Guiana
e-mail: gerardmax@caramail.com

[1] These two schemas are from the book: *Pratique Ophtalmologique pour le Médecin généraliste* M. Gerard, PH Dalens, E Denion, P Huguet, ISBN no 2-9521800-0-8) edited by l'ADOG chapter "Anatomy" written by E. Denion (www.adog973.org).

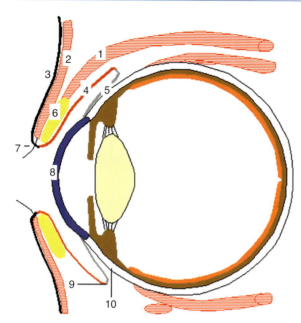

Fig. 7.2 Horizontal section of the eyeball via the fovea centralis (Some extraocular structures are mentioned). *1*, Levator muscle; *2*, Orbicularis oculi muscle; *3*, Eyelid skin; *4*, Palpebral conjunctiva; *5*, Bulbar conjunctiva; *6*, Superior tarsal plate; *7*, Upper eyelid margin; *8*, Cornea; *9*, Conjunctival sac; *10*, Sclera

- The function of the endothelial cells: they permanently pump the water off the cornea so that the cornea is said to be in permanent detergescence.

But all these factors are altered by burns.

The clinical signs of chemical eye burns are the result of the pathophysiology that can be arbitrarily divided into two steps (in reality those two phases are successive but cannot be dissociated):

- Step 1: Destruction of the tissues due to the direct action of the chemical
- Step 2: Corneal reaction to the burn

7.2 Immediate Clinical of the Ocular Chemical Burn

As that for a cardiac arrest, the clinical analysis of the ocular chemical burn is done only after the initiation of an emergency treatment: the eye wash.

The initial clinical signs are the direct consequences of the action of the chemical on the cells, leading to necrosis, and its action on the ocular tissues, which results in the modification of their aspect.

The clinical examination of an ocular chemical burn victim includes all the steps of the ophthalmologic examination: measurement of visual ACUITY, slit lamp, and evaluation of the ocular tonicity.

The patient often suffers from an intense stress, because of the circumstances of the accident:

- Assault, either when the victim knows his/her aggressor in the context of a personal conflict between two people, or on contrary, as a gratuitous violence
- Work accident, when the victim thinks that he/she has made a professional mistake.

Chemical burns generate fear because there are myths and realities about it: a possible evolution of the lesion for a long time after the accident, some important aesthetic sequelae without treatment.

The knowledge of these problems brings in the necessity for the doctor to limit his/her intervention to the field of his/her professional competency, which means that the doctor should, in the initial examination, focus on the clinical analysis without paying too much attention to the particular circumstances.

The ophthalmologic examination may require a local anesthesia by instillation of a collyrium of oxybuprocain type. As that for skin burns, the absence of pain is very often a sign of gravity, but this is not an absolute rule. In ophthalmology and more specifically, concerning burns, there may be no link between the anatomic lesions and the pain.

7.2.1 Initial and Essential Clinical Signs of the Ocular Chemical Burns

There are three initial signs highlighting the ocular chemical burn.

7.2.1.1 The Perilimbal (or Conjunctival) Ischemia

The perilimbal ischemia is the breaking of the conjunctival and episcleral vessels resulting in a plus or minus spread white avascular areas around the edge of the limbus (Fig. 7.3).

7.2 Immediate Clinical of the Ocular Chemical Burn

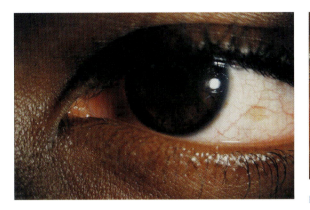

Fig. 7.3 The limbus is the junction between the transparent cornea and the conjunctiva (vascular zone)

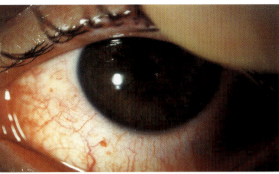

Fig. 7.4 Conjunctival hyperhemia of a benign ocular burn caused by Mancenillier latex, 3 h after accident

The limbus is the anatomic junction between the transparent cornea and the conjunctiva, a tissue in which the vessels circulate. At this level, there would be the limbal stem cells, cells generating the differentiated epithelial cells of the cornea. The essential property of the cornea is transparency. The seriousness of the ocular burn consists in the loss of the corneal transparency. Actually the limbus is a real barrier to the conjunctiva. In the following months, a serious ocular burn will result in the development of a conjunctival cover leading to a loss of vision.

The conjunctival ischemia results from the necrosis of the endothelial cells of the conjunctival and scleral vessels. There is often a blood extravasation so that the conjunctival hemorrhages are often associated to this ischemia.

This ischemia can be trivial, limited to the breaking of the blood flux in only one vessel and not easy to detect because of being hidden in a spread conjunctival hyperemia. The conjunctival hyperemia differs from ischemia. The conjunctival hyperemia is a dilatation of the conjunctival and episcleral vessels. It signifies an inflammation as a reaction to the irritation caused by the chemical burn. It is not a sign of the gravity of the chemical burn (Fig. 7.4).

Ischemia may be major with absence of blood flux over the entire ocular surface, making it look like dead eye (Fig. 7.5).

Conjunctival ischemia is the major sign of chemical burns; the extent of this ischemia is the medium of evaluation of the secondary ability of back growth of the corneal epithelium. Even before the theory of corneal limbal stem cells was mentioned, Hugues had

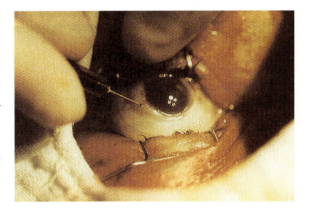

Fig. 7.5 Very serious ocular burn by alkali (12.8% ammonia, pH = 11.5), 1 h 30 min after accident: complete 360° conjunctival ischemia (none of the conjunctival or episcleral vessels are visible)

already found a correlation between the extent of the ischemia and the prognosis of burns.

A burn is very serious with reserved prognosis when ischemia spreads on more than half of the limbal circumference (Fig. 7.6). Most of the times, this ischemia predominates on the lower half of the limbus, because it is where the chemical, in general a liquid, concentrates. It is necessary to emphasize that the maximum quantity of liquid which can cover the surface of the eye is 200 μL.

7.2.1.2 Ulcer of the Cornea

The ulcer of the cornea is the abrasion of the cornea surface, secondary to the epithelial necrosis; it may also alter a deeper layer, the corneal stroma.

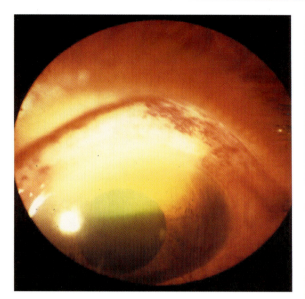

Fig. 7.6 Upper conjunctival ischemia of a serious ocular chemical burn by alkali (12.8% ammonia, pH = 11.5)

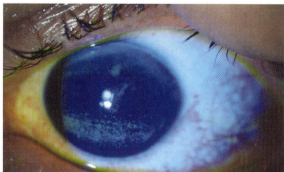

Fig. 7.7 Superficial punctuate keratitis all over the corneal surface, but predominating on the lower part; examination 3 h after burn by a Mancenillier tree

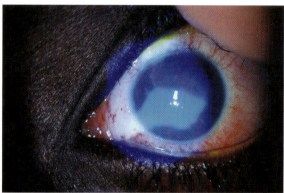

Fig. 7.8 Inferior corneal ulceration displayed by fluorescein with, opposite, a conjunctival ischemia also marked nasally

Its examination follows the instillation of a drop a fluorescein into the conjunctival sac, closure of the eyelids for the fluorescein to spread over all the corneal surface, then ocular wash with physiological saline or by waiting for the natural wash with the tears of the affected eye. Often forgotten, this last element is a factor of misevaluation of the corneal ulcer. A better estimate of the ulcer is obtained by using blue light that highlights the defects of the corneal surface and makes them glow green.

The importance of the ulcer of the cornea enables the estimate of the seriousness of an ocular chemical burn.

It may be benign, limited to a simple superficial punctuate keratitis mostly in the lower part of the palpebral gap, but may also alter the upper part, normally located under the upper eyelid (Fig. 7.7).

The ulcer may be bigger and visible as more or less wide zones in the area of the palpebral gap and mainly in the lower part. These are carved as on a geographic map (Fig. 7.8).

The ulcer is evidently visible when there are some epithelial cells left; these cells will form the edge of the ulcer. In case of a complete ulcer (necrosis of the epithelial cells), it could be difficult for a neophyte to spot it. The image is the same as the one of a corneal surface looking evenly green, like when there is no ulcer ; however, this image remains even after a wash with a normal saline solution.

A complete corneal ulcer is a sign of the seriousness of a burn. The theory of the limbal stem cells may explain that experimental fact. Actually, in that theory, those cells, which are the only ones to regenerate some mature epithelial corneal cells, would be located around the corneal epithelium. Like the conjunctival ischemia, the complete corneal ulcer is an indirect sign of probable destruction of the limbal stem cells. Nevertheless, a complete corneal ulcer or a corneal ulcer that completely releases the optical axis, does not cause any loses of visual acuity.

7.2.1.3 Edema of the Cornea

The edema of the cornea is the diminution or even the complete loss of the corneal transparency (Fig. 7.9).

The edema reveals a serious ocular burn; its importance is correlated with the seriousness of the burn.

7.2 Immediate Clinical of the Ocular Chemical Burn

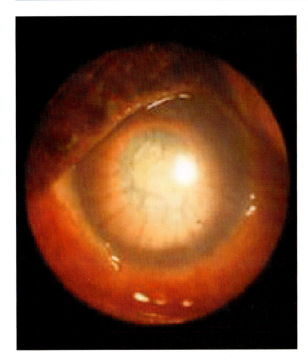

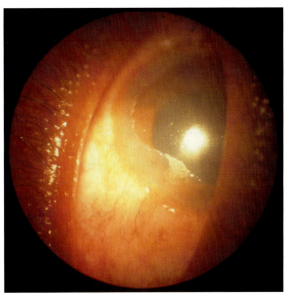

Fig. 7.10 Epithelial necrosis with, under, transparent stroma

Fig. 7.9 Medium edema of the cornea caused by a burn by alkali (12.8% ammonia, pH = 11.5), examination 12 h after accident

The edema may be benign, thus enabling a complete examination of all the structures of the anterior chamber: iris, pupil, and lens. The edema may be medium when it makes the cornea translucent and then only a faded iris can be observed. It may also be important, and then it creates a "porcelain like" cornea, meaning a white cornea, in which none of the structures of the anterior chamber are visible. This stromal edema must not be taken for an epithelial necrosis due to coagulation, which is sometimes present in some specific types of burns. The epithelium with a necrosis can and must be taken off with a cotton wool stick or a scarificator. This epithelium is easy to separate from the eye, in the form of a whitish squame and then lets the transparent stroma to appear (Fig. 7.10).

7.2.2 Roper Hall's Prognostic Classification of the Chemical Eye Burns

A prognostic classification of the chemical eye burn can be based on these three initial signs:

Step	Initial clinical analysis	Prognosis
Grade 1	Epithelial alteration No limbal ischemia	Good
Grade 2	Blurred but visible cornea Lower ischemia on one third of the limbal circumference	Good
Grade 3	Complete loss of the corneal epithelium Stromal blurring preventing the visibility of the iris Ischemia covering one third to half of the limbal circumference	Reserved
Grade 4	Opaque cornea Iris is not visible Major ischemia altering more then half of the limbal circumference	Bad

Fig. 7.11 Roper Hall's Prognostic classification

Hugues classification modified by Roper Hall (Fig. 7.11).

Grades 1 and 2 are classified as benign chemical eye burns. Their prognosis is good and they usually heal within ten days or so.

Grades 3 and 4 are considered as serious chemical eye burns. Their functional and anatomic prognosis is reserved or even bad for grade 4.

Because of a plus or minus long time between the burn and the examination and the possible apparition of late clinical signs, particularly in case of eye burns by bases, it is a common agreement that a next day examination enables a better evaluation of the seriousness of the burn. However, even in the first minutes following the burn, a thorough examination enables a good evaluation of the seriousness of the burn.

7.2.3 The Initial Sketch

All of the ocular clinical signs will be reported on a simple sketch including, at least:

- The extent of the conjunctival ischemia, the evaluation of which is essential for a probable secondary surgery treatment: the autograft of limbus. The accurate measurement of the conjunctival ischemia in the limbal zone is indeed important because the altered zones cannot supply stem cells whereas the superior zones without ischemia can be used as grounds for the sampling of stem cells. Measured in degrees, the extent of this safe region is also important to know if it can be used for its efficiency as a graft as well as to reduce the risk of lack of stem cells for the donor eye. This last point is the reason why a lot of authors limit the recommendation of autograft to unilateral burns and usually prefer the option of the graft of amniotic membrane.
- The ulcer of the cornea. Successive sketches show the evolution of the cicatrization of the epithelium, which is a centripetal phenomenon.

7.2.4 Other Initial Signs of Chemical Eye Burn

The initial clinical examination of an eye burn can also reveal other signs of seriousness:

- Either signs of alteration of the conjunctiva
- Or signs of the intraocular lesions due to the penetration of the chemical into the eye. We shall remind that the penetration of a chemical into the eye is very fast and happens within the first minute after projection (See Sect. 5.16 and Fig. 5.12).

7.2.4.1 Signs of Alteration of the Conjunctiva

We have highlighted above the importance of the accurate evaluation of the zone of conjunctival ischemia on the limbal part because of the probable later necessity of sampling the safe zone.

The evaluation of the conjunctival hurts on the conjunctival zone is also important. Thus, the conjunctival ulcer must be measured like the corneal ulcer which reacts with fluorescein. In general, the conjunctival ulcer corresponds to the zone of ischemia. But the conjunctival ischemia may alter zones with no conjunctival ulcer.

In chemical eye burns, there is always a fast enough conjunctival cicatrization but it may generate some symblepharons. Symblepharons are adherences that develop between the eyelids and the eyeball. They may cause a reduction of the mobility of both eye and eyelids. They are the result of between the bulbar conjunctiva and the palpebral conjunctiva sticking to each other after the cicatrization of the bulbar and palpebral conjunctival ulcers facing each other. It is then necessary to examine with meticulous care the entire surface of the conjunctiva including the conjunctival sacs. Because of the bulbar and palpebral conjunctival ulcers, the prevention of later adherences requires the placement of antisymblepharon rings.

At last, the examination of an eye burn patient aims to search and eliminate any concretion, particularly at the level of the conjunctival sacs. These concretions may help a continuation of the burn, because they are due to precipitations of either the chemical (for instance, lime) or dust projected with the chemical. These concretions result in the gradual decomposition of the compound at the level of the eye.

7.2.4.2 Signs of Intraocular Lesions

When the burn is serious, the initial examination may reveal:

- A Tyndall effect in the anterior chamber. The presence of an intraocular inflammation is a bad prognosis
- The presence of pigments on the inner side of the cornea. Released by the iris, these pigments reveal a high concentration of chemical in the anterior chamber. Except in some very rare cases, such burns result in eye atrophy
- A cataract

But all of these signs also show that the eye reacts to the burn. Actually, they may also appear in a secondary time.

At last, the clinical examination of the eye also requires a measurement of the ocular pressure. The corneal ulcer makes this measurement using an applanation tonometer dangerous (risk of infection). It can now be done with lower risks of infection thanks to the use of an air-puff tonometer. In general, the ocular pressure is normal in the initial step.

7.2.4.3 Extraocular Signs

Most of the times, chemical eye burns are due to projections of chemicals to the face. It is important that the initial clinical analysis mentions the associated clinical signs, as far as the circumstances of the chemical burn often give them a medicolegal interest. These signs may be:

- Palpebral burns
- Face burns, the depth of which is to be estimated as first, second, or third degree. As these hurts are caused by liquid substances, in general, the burns are a little deep but really extended.
- Burns of the lacrymal system. They are uneasy to evaluate, however looking for a stenosis of the lacrymal point or canaliculi is essential. Concerning serious chemical eye burns, a systematic wash of the lacrymal system also enables to check its permeability.
- Burns of the nose mucous membrane, because of the chemical passing through the lacrymal system. It is necessary to do a nasal examination no later than the next day after the accident.
- Burns of the lips and mouth mucous membrane

7.3 Clinical Examination of the Evolution of Chemical Eye Burns

There are two types of evolution.

7.3.1 Benign Ocular Burns

Benign ocular burns are grade 1 and grade 2 ocular burns. They evolve toward healing within 10 days or so. In this case, the epithelium of the cornea centripetally and gradually grows back. Treatments aim to prevent infectious complications and to support cicatrization.

7.3.2 Serious Ocular Burns

Serious ocular burns are grade 3 and grade 4 ocular burns. After primary alteration of the ocular biological tissues by the chemical, some biological reactions of cicatrization develop. As in any cicatrization, there are two phases: the detersion phase to eliminate the altered tissues and the repairing phase. Serious eye burns modify these two phases: they increase the ability of detersion and reduce the ability of reparation. Such a cicatrization then takes several weeks or months until consolidation of the lesions.

7.3.2.1 Complications on the Ocular Surface

Corneal Nonhealing

The absence of corneal cicatrization is illustrated by a recurrent ulcer of the cornea that will first reduce then form again and never heal (Fig. 7.12).

At such a step and every 48 h, there must be a thorough clinical examination of the corneal edema, because it is certainly a cause of the noncicatrization of the cornea. A good illustration of this phenomenon is the image of a roof collapsing because it is supported by a too weak structure. The epithelial

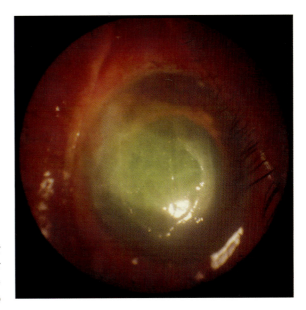

Fig. 7.12 Recurrent ulcer of the cornea after ocular burn by alkali (12.8% ammonia, pH = 11.5)

cells and particularly their basement membrane cannot be supported by a corneal stroma with edema. This clinical notion has a therapeutic interest: the use of anti-inflammatory and corticoid drugs to reduce and eliminate the edema. But these drugs have an inhibitive effect on the back growth of the epithelium, so they must be stopped as soon as the edema reduces, whereas the prescription of medicines facilitating the epithelialization must be increased. On the other hand, the stromal edema is not the only cause of the development of a marginal ulcer. The lack of limbal stem cells is also a primordial element of the evolution of this pathology. The evaluation of the remaining capital of the burnt eye is indirect and rough, and based on the observations of the initial examination. At this stage, while considering the rest of the ocular state, an autograft of limbus or a graft of amniotic membrane can be proposed.

The spontaneous evolution of this type of ulcer is dramatic and within a few weeks results in the conjunctival covering. This phenomena begins in the zone where limbal stem cells are the most insufficient, that is, as a general rule, in the inferior part. It gradually develops over the entire corneal surface and finally results in a complete conjunctiva that is completely covered and a loss of visual function of the damaged eye (Figs. 7.13 and 7.14).

The noncicatrization of the ulcer may also result in a spontaneous puncture of the cornea (Fig. 7.15).

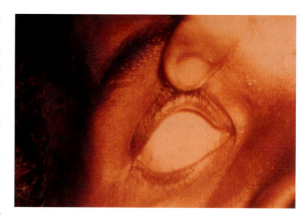

Fig. 7.14 Old conjunctival covering due to eye burn. The patient perceives the light

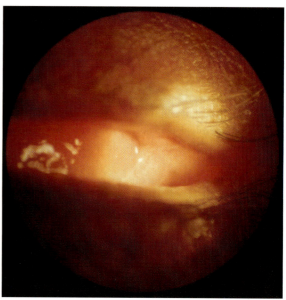

Fig. 7.15 Spontaneous puncture of the cornea after eye burn by alkali (12.8% ammonia, pH = 11.5) with numerous symblepharons completely preventing the opening of the eyelids

Other Complications on the Ocular Surface

There might be other complications on the ocular surface like:

- Abscess of the cornea, which must be systematically prevented by checking the antitetanic vaccination and the prescription of local therapies by antibiotics.
- Symblepharons, which must also be systematically prevented by the installation of a symblepharon

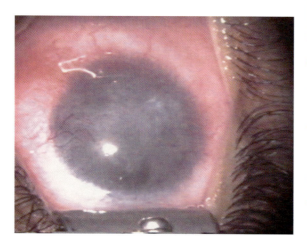

Fig. 7.13 Beginning of a conjunctival covering after eye burn by alkali (12.8% ammonia, pH = 11.5)

ring and/or by releasing them by passing a swab twice a day into the conjunctival sacs. The secondary treatment of symblepharons is far more complex and requires the techniques of reconstruction of the conjunctival sacs via a graft of mouth mucous membrane.

- Ectropium-trichiasis of the burnt eyelids, which very often develops simultaneously with symblepharons and causes a chronic irritation of the ocular surface that may result in some relapsing local infections. This entropium-trichiasis must be treated by surgical techniques including an eversion of the tarsus, associated with an exeresis of the eyelid margin at once as well as an exeresis of the adjacent conjunctiva wearing the ciliated folliculi with trichiasis and suture of a graft of mouth mucous membrane.
  – Healing of the cornea with the following potential consequences:
  – Persistent corneal edema, limiting the visual acuity and mainly reserving the long-term functional, even anatomical, prognosis of this burned eye
  – Corneal leucoma: opaque and white scar (Fig. 7.16) often with an irregular astigmatism and limited visual acuity of this eye
  – Frosted cornea having lost its transparency with, often associated, irregularity of its surface and the peripheral neovessels

7.3.2.2 Endocular Complication

Endocular complications occur in case of a serious burn. They aggravate the already very reserved prognosis of these burns. They may be associated with each other with no preference and may be the following ones:

- Ocular hypertonia, which reveals either a direct lesion of the trabeculum by the chemical, or an inflammatory, reaction due to the burn. Hypertonia usually occurs during the second or third week following the burn. It must be recognized and treated by a topical treatment and a general hypotonizing therapy. It causes or aggravates the corneal edema, which is a limiting factor of the back growth of the corneal epithelium.
- Endocular inflammation. These inflammations usually generate synechia of the iris with the lens, which must be prevented by the instillation of mydriatic and cycloplegic collyrium.
- Cataract: opacity of the lens. It is sometimes visible from the initial examination but, more often, it appears secondarily. It is the consequence of the intensity and the depth of the ocular lesions. It is an element revealing a very bad final prognosis for the burned eye.
- Atrophy of the eye, ultimate evolution, usual and delayed (in the months that follow the accident) for serious chemical eye burns. This eye is obviously no more functional (absence of light perception). It is then necessary, in aesthetic purposes, to make an eviceration or an enucleation (ablation of the contents of the eye or its totality) allowing the implementation of an eye prosthesis. It is then the anatomical loss of the globe.

This chapter is based on the personal experience of the author already published, partially, in articles listed in the bibliography.

Bibliography

Beare, J.D.L.: Eye injuries from assault with chemicals. Br J Ophthalmol **74**, 514–518 (1990)

Branday, J., Arscott, G.D.L., Smoot, E.C., Williams, G.D., Fletcher, P.R.: Chemical burns as assault injuries in Jamaica. Burns **22**, 154–155 (1996)

Burns, F.R., Paterson, C.A.: Chemical injuries: Mechanisms of corneal damage and repair. In: Beuerman, R.W., Crosson, C.E., Kaufman, H.E. (eds.) Healing Processes in the Cornea. Advances in Applied Biotechnology Series, vol. 1, pp. 45–58. Gulf, Houston (1989)

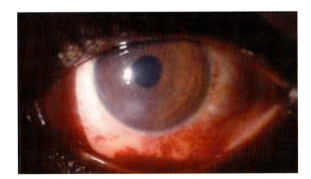

Fig. 7.16 Corneal healing with inferior leucoma post 33% HCl burn

Gérard, M., Merle, H.: Une agression par projection de liquide au visage. Panorama du médecin **4422**, 19 (1996)

Gérard, M., Merle, H., Domenjôd, M., Ayeboua, L., Richer, R., Jallot Sainte Rose, N.: Brûlures oculaires par bases. A propos de 6 cas. Ophtalmologie **10**, 413–417 (1996)

Gérard, M., Merle, H., Chiambaretta, F., Louis, V., Richer, R., Rigal, D.: Technique chirurgicale de l'autotransplantation limbique dans les brûlures oculaires graves récentes. J Fr Ophtalmol **22**(4), 502–506 (1999a)

Gérard, M., Merle, H., Ayeboua, L., Richer, R.: Etude prospective de 3 ans des brûlures oculaires par bases au C.H.U. de Fort de France. J Fr Ophtalmol **22**(8), 834–847 (1999b)

Gérard, M., Louis, V., Merle, H., Josset, P., Menerath, J.M., Blomet, J.: Etude expérimentale sur la pénétration intraoculaire de l'ammoniaque. J Fr Ophtalmol **22**(10), 1047–1053 (1999c)

Gérard, M., Josset, P., Louis, V., Menerath, J.M., Blomet, J., Merle, H.: Existe-il un délai pour le lavage oculaire externe dans le traitement d'une brûlure oculaire par l'ammoniaque. Comparaison de deux solutions de lavage: sérum physiologique et Diphotérine®. J Fr Ophtalmol **23**(5), 449–458 (2000)

Gérard, M., Merle, H., Chiambaretta, F., Rigal, D., Schrage, N.: An amphoteric rinse used in the emergency treatment of a serious ocular burn. Burns **28**(7), 670–673 (2002)

Hugues Jr., W.F.: Alkali burns of the eye. Review of literature and summary of present knowledge. Arch Ophthalmol **35**, 423–449 (1946a)

Hugues Jr., W.F.: Alkali burns of the eye. Clinical and pathological course. Arch Ophthalmol **36**, 189–214 (1946b)

Kuckelkorn, R., Schrage, N., Keller, G., Redbrake, C.: Emergency treatment of chemical and thermal eye burns. Acta Ophthalmol Scand **80**(1), 4–10 (2002)

Lagoutte, F.: Traumatismes et brûlures. In: Rigal, D. (ed.) L'épithélium cornéen. Rapport de la Société Française d'Ophtalmologie, pp. 210–214. Masson, Paris (1993)

Merle, H., Donnio, A., Ayeboua, L., Michel, F., Thomas, F., Ketterle, J., Leonard, C., Josset, P., Gérard, M.: Alkali ocular burns in Martinique (French West Indies). Evaluation of the use of an amphoteric solution as the rinsing product. Burns **31**(2), 205–211 (2005)

Pouliquen, Y., Petroutsos, G.: Brûlures oculaires. In: Encycl. Méd. Chir. Ophtalmologie. Editions techniques. Paris, 21700 C10 (1983)

Ropper-Hall, J.: Thermal and chemical burns. Trans Ophthalmol Soc UK **85**, 634–653 (1965)

Tseng, S.C.G.: Concept and applications of limbal stem cells. Eye **3**(2), 141–157 (1989)

Wagoner, M.D., Kenyon, K.R.: Chemical injuries. In: Shingleton, B.J., Hersh, P.S., Kenyon, K.R., Topping, T.M., Woog, J.J. (eds.) Eye Trauma, pp. 107–114. Mosby, St Louis (1991)

Surgical Therapeutic of Ocular Burns

Harold Merle

8.1 Surgical Treatment of Ocular Burns

Sometimes, the presence of a noisy symptomatology can make the initial clinical examination difficult, although the latter enables to draw up a prognosis and mostly to drive the surgical care. The condition of the cornea is the major element in the definition of the surgical behavior. It is crucial to know whether there is or is not destruction of the limbal stem cells.

8.1.1 Debridement/Excision of the Necrotic Tissues

Same as for local corticotherapy, the goal of excision is to reduce the inflammatory reaction due to the products resulting from the alteration of the necrotic conjunctiva and involved in the detersion of the site. Thus, it limits the production of free oxygenated cytotoxic radicals. It also allows the removal of the caustic material that has stored up in these tissues. The excision must be operated as soon as the eyeball has been rinsed and potential foreign bodies ablated. It consists in the ablation of the necrotic tissues of the eyeball surface. The excision of the conjunctiva and of the subconjunctival tissue must be done up to the superior and inferior fornix when required. Only the necrotic and avascular tissues must be removed until the reach of the tissue layers with safe traffic blood. The scleral tissue, even if ischemic, and the cornea must be respected [1].

8.1.2 Prevention of the Formation of Symblepharons

The prevention of the formation of symblepharons is to be considered in any case of extended burn of the cornea. Several methods are available: the regular release of adherences from the conjunctival sacs with the help of a glass stick or with a swab, which is operated under local anesthesia, the set up of scleral glasses or of polymethyl-methacrylate rings, the use of big diameter bandaging contact lenses [2]. Yamada suggests the installation of gelatine sponges in the conjunctival sac [3].

8.1.3 Tenon's Plastics

In severe ocular burns with complete loss of the limbal vascularization, other than the predictable impossibility of secondary re-epithelialization, there is an immediate risk of necrosis for the anterior segment. In order to restore the limbal circulation and to block the evolution towards a necrosis or an aseptic ulceration, a Tenon's plastics may be realized. It consists in the making of a Tenon's advancement flap located at the level of the limbus [4–8]. The intervention must be realized as soon as the necrotic tissues have been removed. The dissection starts in the equatorial region and continues at the back of the conjunctival sacs. The flaps must be 1–2 mm thick. Their elastic consistency helps their advancement. The flap is sutured to the

H. Merle
Head of the Ophthalmologist,
Department of Ophthalmology,
University Hospital, Fort de France,
Guadeloupe, French Indies
e-mail: harold.merle@chu-fortdefrance.fr

limbus and, at 3 mm at the back, sutured to the sclera by some stitches separated from the resorbable threads. There must be one flap in each dial. The Tenon's capsule is quickly covered with a stratified and even conjunctival epithelium. In more than 80% of the cases, the epithelialization is achieved within less than 20 days and the fornix is then big enough in 60% of the cases [5]. Either because of the thinness of the tissue or because of an insufficient proximal vascularization, the distal end of the flap may sometimes become ischemic. The fluorescein angiography enables the visualization of the ischemia before the development of the necrosis. Tenon's plastics may also be operated later in case of a corneal-scleral ulceration.

This technique facilitates the scleral cicatrization and prevents the formation of scleral ulcers but it does not enable the covering of the corneal surface with a normal phenotype corneal epithelium [8]. It does not completely avoid the development of a conjunctival fibrosis or of symblepharons. The formation of symblepharons, 28% in Kuckelkorn series, is most often recorded within the first three months. This situation may require the realization of a new Tenon's plastics or of a transplant of conjunctiva, nose, or mouth mucous membrane.

8.1.4 The Conjunctival Transplantation

First developed by Thoft, the conjunctival transplantation does not enable the cicatrization of the corneal epithelium [9]. In this field of application, it has been supplanted with the graft of limbal stem cells. However, it is still advised as a factor of restoration of the conjunctival sacs after they have been reshaped by cicatricial fibrosis. The conjunctiva is the best graft to use because it provides a basement membrane as well as mucous cells. Obviously, this special graft is available only if one eye has been damaged and convincing the patient that their safe eye must be operated may be hard work. The sample, about 1.5 × 2 cm big, is taken from the upper bulbar conjunctiva of the safe eye. An injection of lidocaine helps the separation of the conjunctiva from the subconjunctival tissue. After the excision of the cicatricial zones, the graft is positioned and sutured to the bare sclera. In case of rebuilding of the fornix, the graft must be sutured to the tarsal conjunctiva and kept in contact with the subjacent tissues.

Usually used in surgery of the retina, a Silastic® band can be placed into the conjunctival sac and maintained with two transcutaneous sutures. This perfectly maintains the graft to the bottom of the fornix and prevents the development of synechia.

8.1.5 Transplantation of Buccal and Nasal Mucosa

The graft of buccal mucosa is usually sampled from the posterior side of the upper or lower lip. It is much thinner than the jugal graft. The sampling zone is infiltrated with Xylocaine® adrenaline. The incision is located at least 1 cm at the back of the lower lip edge. The dissection is made using scissors or a bistoury blade and must be as least deep as possible. The hemostasis is cautiously realized in order to prevent any hurt of the nervous structures, which are the generators of the sensitivity of the lip. There is no suture. A 1-week local treatment is prescribed. The cicatrization should take 2–8 days. The surface of such a graft is 1.5 cm wide and 4 cm long. Its retraction is about 1/3. The buccal mucosa is thinned using scissors, at the expense of its posterior side [10]. Some complications correlated with the sampling of buccal mucosa have been described: hurt of the opening of the parotid duct, scars under mucosa, and contractures. The buccal mucosa may be used for the treatment of a symblepharon, a trichiasis, a distichiasis, an entropion, or a keratinized zone of the conjunctiva or of the palpebral margin.

The transplant of nasal mucosa was first prescribed by Naumann for the treatment of severe and bilateral conjunctival mucous shortages. In a study of 24 patients including 16 victims of a severe eye burn with symblepharons, Naumann has observed an improvement of the condition of the ocular surface in all of the cases. He has then concluded that the transplantation of nasal mucosa is better than the transplant of buccal mucosa. When the ocular damage is bilateral, the transplant of nasal mucosa would be perfectly recommended [11]. The nasal cavities are examined with an endoscope in order to find the zone to be sampled. The graft of nasal mucosa is taken from the septum, from the lower or medium turbinates. Under endoscopy and after local anesthesia, the anterior part of the turbinates is usually sampled. A hemostasis is cautiously operated and a gauze plugging of the cavity is set up. This latter will be removed on the day following the operation. There is a risk of atrophic rhinitis. The sample of nasal mucosa is from 4 to 15 cm^2 big and about 1–2 mm thick. The nasal mucosa is sutured to the sclera and to the tarsal conjunctiva by separated stitches of resorbable thread. A silicone strip may be used to maintain and stick the graft to the conjunctival sacs, for about 1 month. A 1-week local therapy by antibiotics is prescribed and a local therapy by corticoids for several weeks. The advantage of the transplant of nasal mucosa is the opportunity to sample big size grafts and the transplantation of intra-epithelial mucus cells. It thus enables the restoration of the mucous constituent of the lacrymal film.

Kuckelkorn does not advise the practice of this intervention during the critical phase of the burn but prefers the Tenon's plastics [12].

8.1.6 The Transplantation of Limbus

Proposed by Schermer and developed by Tseng, the theory of the limbal stem cells (LSC) is the basis of the transplant of limbus [13, 14]. The corneal epithelium quickly regenerates, from undifferentiated LSC located in the basement layers of the limbus. LSC divide and generate some differentiated epithelial cells: the amplifying transitional cells, which migrate toward the center of the cornea in order to form a basement foundation with intense mitotic activity in this location. During various successive cellular cycles, the amplifying transitional cells progressively acquire the phenotypic characteristics of the corneal epithelial cells. These then vertically migrate with a decreasing mitotic activity, and mute into hyperdifferentiated cells at the surface of the cornea. Then, they disappear and therefore desquamate the lacrymal film.

The syndrome of LSC deficiency is characterized by the invasion of the corneal surface by a conjunctival type of epithelium. In this epithelium, the presence of calciform cells is phatognomic of the syndrome of LSC deficiency. The latter is highlighted by a late and bad quality reepithelialization and a superficial and stromal "neovascularization." The grading of ocular burns such as proposed by Dua and Wagoner are based on the importance of the LSC deficit [15, 16].

8.1.6.1 Exeresis of the Conjunctival Pannus

This technique has been introduced by Dua and others [17]. It consists in the exeresis of the conjunctival pannus that is invading the cornea and also enables the development of the corneal epithelium and its migration toward the damaged corneal surface. It is practiced when the conjunctival proliferation covers the cornea by more than 2 mm. The mechanical debridement by scraping is processed from the center toward the edge until 5–7 mm at the back of the limbus. In a series of 14 patients studied for about 8 months, there has been a covering surface by the corneal epithelium. Longer-term results have not been mentioned. This method is an interesting option in comparison with the limbal transplantation when the damage alters a small zone or when the transplantation cannot be operated.

8.1.6.2 The Limbus Autograft

The limbus autograft is the first class technique for the treatment of a destruction of the corneal limbus and the so generated complications [18]. This conjunctival and limbal transplantation technique was described by Kenyon and Tseng in 1989 [19]. It treats the unilateral limbal deficiencies when one eye can be used as a contralateral safe donor. All of the conjunctival pannus covering the cornea is taken off beyond the limbus on about 3 mm. The dissection goes from the cornea – as a starting point – toward the conjunctiva [64]. The graft is sampled from an incision into the cornea, made 1 mm before the limbus. The dissection makes a surgical formation of tunnel from about 2 mm at the back of the limbus. In order to prevent the donor eye from a limbal deficiency, the graft must not be longer than 180° [20]. The sample is sutured to the receiving site by some separated stitches of 10/0 nylon thread to the cornea and by some resorbable 8/0 thread to the conjunctiva.

The limbus autograft requires a good quality corneal reepithelialization for 75–100% patients and the constitution of a barrier preventing the neovascular cicatricial phenomena of conjunctival origin [18, 21, 22]. The date of intervention from the date of burn is a subject of argument. Most authors consider that it is better to wait several months for the inflammatory reaction to decrease. However, some authors recommend an earlier intervention, before the development of complications due to the LSC deficit [16, 23].

8.1.6.3 The Limbus Allograft

The limbus allograft has the same goal as the autograft [24]. The limbus allograft is operated in case of extended limbal lesions whether they are bilateral or unilateral on a unique eye. The tissue is sampled from a corneal graft or from an eye kept by a bank of tissues. The graft must be sampled within 24 h because the lifetime of LSC in a preservation milieu is not well known [25]. The sample must fulfill the requirements of a transfixion keratoplasty. It results from two concentric trepanations: one located 1 mm before the limbus and the other 2 mm at the back. The dissection of a lamella goes from the corneal side – as a starting point – to the conjunctiva. The dimension of the sample relates to the limbal destruction. It may cover all of the limbal edge (360°). It is sutured to the receiving cornea by some separated stitches of 10/0 nylon threads and to the conjunctiva by some resorbable 8/0 threads. The sample may be more scarcely taken from a living donor who is a relative of the victim [26]. The limbus allograft improves the condition of the ocular surface in more than 50% cases. It also improves the prognosis of a secondary penetrating keratoplasty [17, 20, 27]. There is a major risk of graft rejection and this requires a prolonged immunosuppression. The therapy by corticoids and the cyclosporine are prescribed as local and general treatments. A matching HLA type between donor and recipient should lower the rejection risk, but it yet requires an immunosuppressive therapy [26, 28]. The limbus autograft combined with a transplantation of amniotic membrane enables the restoration of the corneal epithelium of normal phenotype [29].

8.1.7 The Transplantation of Amniotic Membrane

Used for ocular burns as soon as 1947 by Sorsby [30], the amniotic membrane is a tissue located at the interface of the placenta and the amniotic fluid. It is constituted of an unstratified epithelium, a basement lamina, and an avascular mesenchyma. The amniotic membrane facilitates the reepithelialization by reducing the inflammatory and cicatricial reaction [31]. It helps the migration of the epithelial cells and the adhesion of the basement cells [32]. It behaves as an actual replacing basement membrane and facilitates the phenotypic epithelial expression. As it is not doted of class II HLA antigens, the amniotic membrane cannot be rejected. The amniotic membrane used for transplantation comes from a placenta taken from a delivery without cesarean operation in order to reduce the risk of bacterial contamination. It is preserved frozen at a −80° temperature. The amniotic membrane must fulfill the same sanitary security norms as a transfixion keratoplasty. The sample of amniotic membrane is sutured, with its epithelial side upwards, to the deepithelialized cornea by some separated 10/0 nylon stitches. Several layers may be layered over each other. The amniotic membrane is covered by the corneal epithelium, integrated to the stroma then resorbed. It can be used for the reflection of the conjunctival sacs after exeresis of the symblepharons [32, 33]. The preoperatory application of 0.04% mitomycin C for 5 min before the positioning of the amniotic membrane would reduce the conjunctival inflammation and improve the depth of the conjunctival sacs and the quality of the lacrymal film [34]. The current trend is to practice the transplantation of amniotic membrane early enough, during the precocious phase of the burn. The reepithelialization would reach more than 80% within 15 days, the visual acuity would improve in 77% cases, and the symblepharons would be rare [35]. Even when the transplantation is practiced later, there are some good results [36].

The transplantation of amniotic membrane does not suffice for the treatment of a severe LSC deficiency due to a burn [37]. In such a case, it needs to be associated with an LSC transplantation. The amniotic membrane is first sutured to the deepithelialized cornea and the limbal graft is set astride the edge of the amniotic membrane [38]. The cicatrization of the corneal epithelium is completed for 75–100% cases within 3 weeks when the LSC deficit is incomplete and for 70% cases when the deficit is complete [39, 40].

8.1.8 Keratoplasties

8.1.8.1 Big Diameter Transfixion Keratoplasty

An 11–12 mm diameter transfixion keratoplasty (TK) provides a double advantage: that of an optic or architectonic keratoplasty and that of an intake of LSC guaranteeing the cicatrization of the corneal epithelium [41, 42]. It can be operated either in the precocious or in the cicatricial phase of severe burns. The big diameter TK has a high risk of rejection, which alters its results. It is preferable to replace it with a preliminary LSC transplantation followed by a usual diameter TK.

8.1.8.2 The Usual Diameter Transfixion Keratoplasty

Burns can cause an edema due to a toxic necrosis of the endothelial cells, an opacification of the corneal stroma, and a thinning of the stroma, which generates an important irregular astigmatism. The aim of the TK is to restore the corneal transparency.

Most of the time, the sampling of cornea is operated by in situ excision. Donors are selected according to criteria defined by the associations of cornea banks, who also assume the quality control, the preservation, and the distribution of the samples. The first step of intervention consists in trepanning the graft to a diameter close to 8 mm. The recipient cornea is then trepanned to a slightly smaller diameter. The most used is the Hessburg–Barron vacuum corneal trephine. The sample is sutured to the recipient cornea by separated stitches and/or by a continuous suture. The postoperatory treatment includes a corticoid collyrium coupled with an antibiotic collyrium prescribed for 1–2 years. Overall about 10%, the risk of rejection is higher for chemical burns, especially because of the frequency and the importance of the stromal neovascularization of the recipient cornea [43–45].

A TK does not provide any LSC; therefore, it does not suffice to treat extended limbal ischemia. It must be coupled with a limbus transplantation [46].

A TK can be practiced in the same operatory step as a limbus allograft. The intervention begins with a limbal peritectomy, followed by the TK [47]. However, the epithelial cicatrization and the corneal transparency are better when the TK is secondarily realized (from 1 to 13 months). The endothelial rejection is less important too: 0% against 53% for a transplantation occurring in the first month [18].

An auto-TK coupled with a limbus autograft may exceptionally be practiced as illustrated in Figs. 8.1–8.4.

This is the case of a monophtalmic left eye patient wounded by a grade 4 burn due to a strong base. Two TK have not succeeded because of successive rejections. The visual acuity of the left eye was reduced to a good localization of the light. The cornea was white,

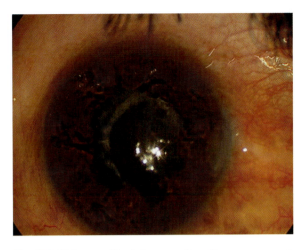

Fig. 8.1 Right eye. No light perception. Presurgery aspect. Clear cornea, calm anterior chamber, old posterior synechia, extracapsular surgical aphakia. Normal ocular pressure

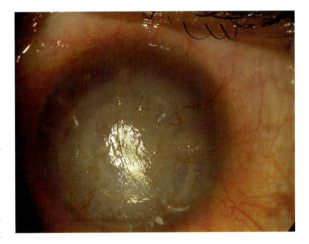

Fig. 8.2 Left eye. Presurgery aspect. Visual acuity reduced to a good localization of the light. White cornea, ulcerated and neovascularized. Complete limbus deficiency related to a 360° destruction of the limbus

ulcerated, and neovascularized. There was a complete limbus deficiency. The right eye had not been functioning since childhood because of a closed contusion. In the same operatory step, we have sampled from the right eye: the cornea (8 mm trepanation) and the limbus over 360°. After the ablation of the conjunctival pannus covering the limbus and the cornea of the left eye, we have transplanted the cornea and the limbus, which had previously been sampled from the left eye.

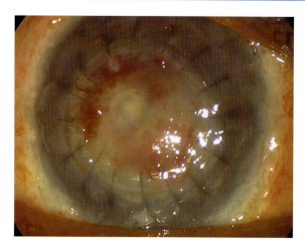

Fig. 8.3 Right eye. One month postsurgery. White left cornea sutured with 16 separated stitches of 10/0 nylon

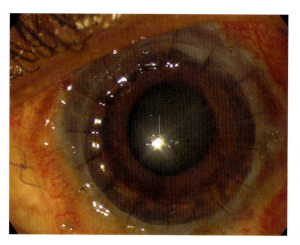

Fig. 8.4 Left eye. One month postsurgery. Clear right cornea sutured with 16 separated stitches of 10/0 nylon. 360° limbus autograft taken from right eye and sutured with 8 separated stitches of 10/0 nylon on the cornea and with 8 separated stitches of 8/0 vicryl on the conjunctiva

8.1.8.3 The Deep Lamellar Keratoplasty

The deep lamellar keratoplasty (DLK) consists in transplanting the stroma and the epithelium of the graft while preserving the Descemet membrane and the endothelium of the recipient. It is used to treat corneal burns in which the Descemet membrane and the endothelium have been spared. The graft is sampled and preserved in the same conditions as the graft used for a TK. The operation begins with an 8 mm trepanation of the graft, followed by a non-transfixing 75% trepanation of the thinnest part of the recipient's cornea. A dissection enables the ablation of the epithelium and of the anterior and medium stroma. An injection of air into the posterior stroma helps to loosen the Descemet membrane and therefore facilitates its exeresis. The Descemet membrane of the sample is removed with the use of a pincer and the graft is sutured to the recipient cornea in the same manner as when practicing a TK.

As the endothelium is not grafted, the risk of endothelial rejection is nil. Yao records the results achieved by limbus autografts combined with DLP for 34 patients with sequelae due to unilateral corneal burns. All patients were operated at least 6 months after the burn. All had normal lacrymal secretion. The DLP was practiced at the same operatory time as the limbus autograft. The operation begins with the DLP, followed by the limbus autograft. In 30 cases, there is an improvement of the visual acuity and the central corneal transparency is restored for 29 patients [48]. The series of Fogla includes seven eyes. Very good results are also noticed: improvement of the visual acuity for 85% cases and a 4/10 average postoperatory visual acuity [49]. The practice of a DLP with limbus autograft does not require any immunosuppressive therapy. In comparison with TK, the risk of failure is lower even when the cornea is highly neovascularized [49].

8.1.8.4 The Big Diameter Lamellar Keratoplasty

The big diameter LK was first introduced in the year 2000 by Vajpayee [50] for a use in the surgical treatment of sequelae due to corneal burns. Vajpayee has recorded the results of nine ocular operations. The intervention begins with a conjunctival peritectomy over 360°. The conjunctiva is reclined backwards. The recipient cornea is trepanned to a 12–13 mm diameter and to a 300 μm depth. The lamellar graft is sampled via a trepanation at 1.5 mm back to the limbus in order to include LSC. It is then sutured by 24 10/0 nylon stitches. Despite the limbus allograft, no immunosuppressive therapy has been prescribed. The operation was practiced about 30 months after the occurrence of the burn. Results are recorded after a 7.4 month observation. The visual acuity has improved in six cases. No recurrence of the corneal neovascularization and no rejection have been noticed. The big diameter LK provides LSC and enables to get a steady reepithelialized ocular surface. It is recommended when the deep layers of the cornea have been spared by the burn [50].

8.1.8.5 The Keratoplasty with Architectonic Goal

The keratoplasty with architectonic goal aims to fulfill the loss of corneal substance, which is the origin of a perforation of the eyeball. It is rarely recommended and, most of the time, it is practiced in emergency. It is always necessary to search for an LSC deficiency. The type of keratoplasty to practice depends on the size, the depth, and the site of the lesion. It may be a central TK, an eccentric TK, a central or peripheral DLK.

8.1.9 The Transplantation of Cultivated Limbal Epithelial Cells

The autotransplantation of cultivated limbal epithelial cells to an amniotic membrane is a recent technique. It has been developed by Tsai in Taiwan [51]. A 1 × 2 mm fragment of limbal epithelium is sampled from the safe eye. It is then cultivated for 3 weeks on an amniotic membrane. The epithelial tissue is grafted with the amniotic membrane to the recipient cornea after excision of the fibrovascular tissue. The same technique of culture is used by Shimazaki for allografts. He records the results of 13 cases of limbal epithelial cell allografts, 2 of which have been practiced after sequelae of chemical burns with complete limbal deficiency. The global rate of epithelialization is 46.2%. For the two cases of burns of the research, there is a resulting epithelialization of corneal type after 16 and 22 days, and the visual acuity has clearly improved [52]. Nakamura describes the case of a severe burn on which a transplantation of cultivated epithelial limbal cells was practiced 4 years after the trauma. Two days after the transplantation, the cornea is cicatrized and covered by limbal cells. After 8 months, the condition of the corneal surface is stable and the visual acuity is excellent [53]. Sangwan records 15 cases of TK practiced after transplantation of limbal epithelial cells. After 8 months, the cicatrization is steady for 93% patients and the visual acuity is over 3/10 in eight cases. For this author, the short-term prognosis of a TK after transplantation of cultivated epithelial limbal cells is good [54].

8.1.10 Keratoprosthesis

Keratoprosthesis is the last surgical recourse for the cases of bilateral corneal cecity, when transfixion keratoplasties and transplantations of limbal stem cells can no more be achieved. Keratoprosthesis are made of two elements: a central transparent optic part and a support that provides its fixing onto the cornea. The support can either be synthetic or biologic. Developed by Strampelli in the 1960s, the odonto keratoprosthesis uses the root of a tooth. Although it is uneasy to set up, it is still up to date because its results are sometimes encouraging [55]. More recently, fluorocarbons have been used [56]. The structure of these polymers is similar to a micro fishnet that can be colonized by the corneal stroma. There are numerous types of keratoprosthesis, but none of them has proved to be better than the others. Complications are frequent and dominated by expulsion. This is tragic and irreversible because it is coupled with a necrosis of the cornea, which is followed by an atrophy of the eyeball. The occurrence of a retroprosthetic membrane seems to be more frequent in the cases of burns. Among other complications, there are severe ocular hypertony, endophthalmies, necrosis of the adjacent tissues, retinal detachment, eyeball atrophy. Among 17 cases of keratoprosthesis operated after chemical burns, the visual acuity is lower than 1/10 for 36% after 2 years and for 75% cases after 5 years [57].

8.2 Surgical Treatment of Eyelid Burns

The eyelid skin is the thinnest of the whole human body. Hypodermis has no lipidic structures, replaced with a more or less fibrous subcutaneous fascia. 3rd-grade burns damage the derma and the orbicularis occuli. Deep 2nd-grade and 3rd-grade burns cause major retractions with palpebral eversion and permanent nonocclusion. These phenomena of retraction of the skin and orbicular level are more important in the cases of extended facial burns, in which there is also the retraction of the facial tissues surrounding the eyelids.

8.2.1 Surgical Treatment in the Critical Phase

If eschars occur, a precocious excision-transplantation may be required to facilitate detersion and prevent superinfection. It helps the fight against retraction. Most of the time, the transplantation is a fine dermic-hypodermic transplantation, which has the advantage of requiring less subjacent vascularization than a transplantation of complete skin [58]. When retraction is important, a tarsorrhaphy may be operated [59]. However, this alters the patient's eyesight and makes the surveillance of the eyeball more difficult. The transplantation remains necessary and the tarsorrhaphy may cause damages on the eyelid margin: unevenness, loss of substance, trichiasis, and damages of the lacrymal meatus. A tarsorrhaphy without avivement of the palpebral margins enables a temporary occlusion [60]. The damage of the lacrymal meatus and of the canaliculi may require to set up silicone plugs or either mono or bicanaliculonasal catheters, to prevent a secondary stenosis [61].

8.2.2 Surgical Treatment in the Sequelar Phase

Although the treatment has been properly achieved, including precocious dermic-epidermic transplantations, some burns may complicate with important retraction. Considering a possible softening of the scar within the first 6 months, waiting such a time for the start of the repairing is quite usual when there is no threat for the eyeball. The principle of surgical rebuilding is to completely release the cicatricial zones and to set up a big enough skin transplantation to compensate the loss of substance [62]. It is better to begin with the upper eyelid. The two eyelids of the same eye should never be operated in the same operatory time. It is necessary to reach a supercorrection and a superocclusion. The aesthetic unity of the eyelid should be respected. The incision spreads from one canthus to the other, with a wide overrunning. In height, the upper eyelid spreads from the eyelid margin to the eyebrow and the lower eyelid from the eyelid margin to the palpebraljugal fissure. The mobile part of the upper eyelid (pretarsal part between eyelash and eyelid crease) is extended by fine dermic-epidermic grafts. The immobile part of the upper eyelid requires transplantations of complete skin. The rebuilding of the lower eyelid is made via transplantations of complete skin. The complete skin graft is thicker, with a lower retraction potential (about 10%) and a color closer to normal skin. The grafts of complete skin are perforated and maintained by a bolster. It is taken off on the 6th day after operation. The dermic-epidermic grafts are sampled from the anterior side of the thigh and the grafts of complete skin from the retroarticular area. The presence of retractile scars at the level of the canthus may require Shaped in Z plasties or plasties of bits. The eyebrows may be rebuilt by transplanting some scalp. The absence of eyelash is best repaired by blepharopigmentation or make up. The permanent results are estimated from the 6th month after operation. The use of bits is only recommended for the most severe type of palpebral burns when there is a subjacent vascular deficiency. They are thicker than the grafts and only enable to achieve a less functional and less aesthetic result [63].

8.3 Conclusion

The prognosis of severe types of ocular burns clearly improved during the last decade thanks to a better knowledge of the physiology of the corneal epithelium. The surgical techniques aiming to restore the damaged limbal stem cells have notably improved the prognosis of severe corneal burns. The future of the surgical care depends on the introduction and development of techniques of cellular therapy. These techniques should enable the in vitro culture of limbal stem cells, sampled from the patient's or from a donor's body, and the transplantation of these cells to the damaged zones in a secondary time.

References

1. Reim, M.: The results of ischemia in chemical injuries. Eye **6**, 376–380 (1992); Reim, M., Kuckelkorn, R.: Chemical and thermal lesions in the orbital region. Bull. Soc. Belge Ophtalmol. **245**, 21–28 (1992); Reim, M., Teping, C.: Surgical procedures in the treatment of most severe eye burns. Acta. Ophthalmol. Scand. **67**, 47–54 (1989).

References

2. Dunnebier, E.A., Kok, J.H.: Treatment of an alkali burn induced symblepharon with a megasoft bandage lens. Cornea **12**, 8–9 (1993)
3. Yamada, M., Sano, Y., Watanabe, A., Mashima, Y.: Preventing symblepharon formation with a gelatin sponge in the eye of a patient with an alkali burn. Am J Ophthalmol **123**(4), 552–554 (1997)
4. Teping, C., Reim, M.: Tenoplasty as a new surgical principle in the early treatment of the most severe chemical eye burns. Klin Monatsbl Augenheilkd **194**, 1–5 (1989)
5. Reim, M., Overkamping, B., Kuckelkorn, R.: Two years experience with Tenon-plasty. Ophthalmologe **89**, 534–540 (1992)
6. Reim, M., Teping, C.: Surgical procedures in the treatment of most severe eye burns. Acta Ophthalmol Scand **67**, 47–54 (1989)
7. Kuckelkorn, R., Redbrake, C., Reim, M.: Tenoplasty: A new surgical approach for the treatment of severe eye burns. Ophthalmic Surg Lasers **28**, 105–110 (1997)
8. Kuckelkorn, R., Schrage, N., Reim, M.: Treatment of severe eyes burns by tenoplasty. Lancet **345**, 657–658 (1995)
9. Thoft, R.A.: Conjunctival transplantation. Arch Ophthalmol **95**, 1425–1427 (1977)
10. Shore, J.W., Foster, C.S., Westfall, C.T., Rubin, P.A.: Results of buccal mucosal grafting for patients with medically controlled ocular cicatricial pemphigoid. Ophthalmology **99**, 383–395 (1992)
11. Naumann, G.O., Lang, G.K., Rummelt, V., Wigand, M.E.: Autologous nasal mucosa transplantation in severe bilateral conjunctival mucus deficiency syndrome. Ophthalmology **97**, 1011–1017 (1990)
12. Kuckelkorn, R., Schrage, N., Redbrake, C., Kottek, A., Reim, M.: Autologous transplantation of nasal mucosa after severe chemical and thermal eye burns. Acta Ophthalmol Scand **74**, 442–448 (1996)
13. Schermer, A., Galvin, S., Sun, T.T.: Differentiation-related expression of a major 64K corneal keratin in vivo and in culture suggests limbal location of corneal epithelial stem cells. J Cell Biol **103**, 49–62 (1986)
14. Tseng, S.C.: Concept and application of limbal stem cells. Eye **3**, 141–157 (1989)
15. Dua, H.S., King, A.J., Joseph, A.: A new classification of ocular surface burns. Br J Ophthalmol **85**, 1379–1383 (2001)
16. Wagoner, M.D.: Chemical injuries of the eye: Current concepts in pathophysiology and therapy. Surv Ophthalmol **41**, 275–313 (1997)
17. Dua, H.S., Gomes, J.A.P., Singh, A.: Corneal epithelial wound healing. Br J Ophthalmol **78**, 401–408 (1994)
18. Shimazaki, J., Shimmura, S., Tsubota, K.: Donor source affects the outcome of ocular surface reconstruction in chemical or thermal burns of the cornea. Ophthalmology **111**, 38–44 (2004)
19. Kenyon, K.R., Tseng, S.C.G.: Limbal autograft transplantation for ocular surface disorders. Ophthalmology **96**, 709–723 (1989)
20. Holland, J.H., Schwartz, G.S.: The evolution of epithelial transplantation for severe ocular surface disease and a proposed classification system. Cornea **15**, 549–556 (1996)
21. Rao, S.K., Rajagopal, R., Sitalakshmi, G., Padmanabhan, P.: Limbal allografting from related live donors for corneal surface reconstruction. Ophthalmology **106**, 822–828 (1999)
22. Frucht-Pery, J., Siganos, C.S., Solomon, A., Scheman, L., Brautbar, C., Zauberman, H.: Limbal cell autograft transplantation for severe ocular surface disorders. Graefes Arch Clin Exp Ophthalmol **236**, 582–587 (1998)
23. Morgan, S., Murray, A.: Limbal autotransplantation in the acute and chronic phases of severe chemical injuries. Eye **10**, 349–354 (1996)
24. Tsai, R.J., Tseng, S.C.: Human allograft limbal transplantation for corneal surface reconstruction. Cornea **13**, 389–400 (1994)
25. Tan, D.T., Ficker, L.A., Buckley, R.J.: Limbal transplantation. Ophthalmology **103**, 29–36 (1996)
26. Rao, S.K., Rajagopal, R., Sitalakshmi, G., Padmanabhan, P.: Limbal autografting: Comparison of results in the acute and chronic phases of ocular surface burns. Cornea **18**, 164–171 (1999)
27. Theng, J.T., Tan, D.T.: Combined penetrating keratoplasty and limbal allograft transplantation for severe corneal burns. Ophthalmic Surg Lasers **28**, 765–768 (1997)
28. Ozdemir, O., Tekeli, O., Ornek, K., Arslanpençe, A., Yalçindag, N.F.: Limbal autograft and allograft transplantations in patients with corneal burns. Eye **18**, 241–248 (2004)
29. Espana, E.M., Grueterich, M., Ti, S.E., Tseng, S.C.: Phenotypic study of a case receiving a keratolimbal allograft and amniotic membrane for total stem cell deficiency. Ophthalmology **110**, 481–486 (2003)
30. Sorsby, A., Simmonds, H.: Amniotic membrane graft in caustic burns of the eye (burns of second degree). Br J Ophthalmol **31**, 409–418 (1947)
31. Hao, Y., Ma, D.H., Hwang, D.G., et al.: Identification of antiangiogenic and antiinflammatory proteins in human amniotic membrane. Cornea **19**, 348–352 (2000)
32. Tseng, S.C., Prabhasawat, P., Lee, S.H.: Amniotic membrane transplantation for conjunctival surface reconstruction. Am J Ophthalmol **124**, 765–774 (1997)
33. Solomon, A., Pires, R.T., Tseng, S.C.: Amniotic membrane transplantation after extensive removal of primary and recurrent pterygia. Ophthalmology **108**, 449–460 (2001)
34. Tseng, S.C., Di Pascuale, M.A., Liu, D.T., Gao, Y.Y., Baradaran-Raffi, A.: Intraoperative mitomycin C and amniotic membrane transplantation for fornix reconstruction in severe cicatricial ocular surface diseases. Ophthalmology **112**, 896–903 (2005)
35. Meller, D., Pires, R.T., Mack, R.J., et al.: Amniotic membrane transplantation for acute chemical or thermal burns. Ophthalmology **107**, 980–990 (2000)
36. Ucakhan, O.O., Koklu, G., Firat, E.: Nonpreserved human amniotic membrane transplantation in acute and chronic chemical eye injuries. Cornea **21**, 169–172 (2002)
37. Hanada, K., Shimazaki, J., Shimurra, S., et al.: Multilayered amniotic membrane transplantation for severe ulceration of the cornea and sclera. Am J Ophthalmol **131**, 324–3311 (2001)
38. Stoiber, J., Muss, W.H., Pohla-Gubo, G., Ruckhofer, J., Grabner, G.: Histopathology of human corneas after amniotic membrane and limbal stem cell transplantation for severe chemical burn. Cornea **21**, 482–489 (2002)
39. Shimazaki, J., Yang, H.Y., Tsubota, K.: Amniotic membrane transplantation for ocular surface reconstruction in patients with chemical and thermal burns. Ophthalmology **104**, 2068–2076 (1997)

40. Gomes, J.A., Dos Santos, M.S., Cunha, M.C., Mascaro, V.L., Barros, J.N., De Sousa, L.B.: Amniotic membrane transplantation for partial and total limbal stem cell deficiency secondary to chemical burn. Ophthalmology 110, 466–473 (2003)
41. Redbrake, C., Buchal, V., Reim, M.: Keratoplasty with a scleral rim after most severe eye burns. Klin Monastsbl Augenheilkd 208, 145–151 (1996)
42. Kuckelkorn, R., Keller, G., Redbrake, C.: Long-term results of large diameter keratoplasties in the treatment of severe chemical and thermal eye burns. Klin Monatsbl Augenheilkd 218, 542–552 (2001)
43. Beekhuis, W.H.: Current clinician's opinions on risk factors in corneal grafting. Cornea 14, 39–42 (1995)
44. Mattax, J.B., Mc Culley, J.P.: Corneal surgery following corneal burns. Int Ophthalmol Clin 28, 76–82 (1988)
45. Brown, S.I., Bloomfield, S.E., Pearce, D.B.: Follow-up report on transplantation of the alkali burned cornea. Am J Ophthalmol 77, 538–542 (1974)
46. Zieske, J.D.: Perpetuation of stem cells in the eye. Eye 8, 163–169 (1994)
47. Tsubota, K., Toda, I., Saito, H., Shinozaki, N., Shimazaki, J.: Reconstruction of the corneal epithelium by limbal allograft transplantation for severe ocular surface disorders. Ophthalmology 102, 1486–1496 (1995)
48. Yao, Y.F., Zhang, B., Zhou, P., Jiang, J.K.: Autologous limbal grafting combined with deep lamellar keratoplasty in unilateral eye with severe chemical or thermal burn at late stage. Ophthalmology 109, 2011–2017 (2002)
49. Fogla, R., Padmanabhan, P.: Deep anterior lamellar keratoplasty combined with autologous limbal stem cell transplantation in unilateral severe chemical injury. Cornea 24, 421–425 (2005)
50. Vajpayee, R.B., Thomas, S., Sharma, N., Dada, T., Tabin, G.C.: Large-diameter lamellar keratoplasty in severe ocular alkali burns: A technique of stem cell transplantation. Ophthalmology 107(9), 1765–1768 (2000)
51. Tsai, R.J., Li, L.M., Chen, J.K.: Reconstruction of damaged corneas by transplantation of autologous limbal epithelial cells. N Engl J Med 343, 86–93 (2000)
52. Shimazaki, J., Aiba, M., Goto, E., Kato, N., Shimmura, S., Tsubota, K.: Transplantation of human limbal epithelium cultivated on amniotic membrane for the treatment of severe ocular surface disorders. Ophthalmology 109, 1285–1290 (2002)
53. Nakamura, T., Inatomi, T., Sotozono, C., Koizumi, N., Kinoshita, S.: Successful primary culture and autologous transplantation of corneal limbal epithelial cells from minimal biopsy for unilateral severe ocular surface disease. Acta Ophthalmol Scand 82, 468–471 (2004)
54. Sangwan, V.S., Matalia, H.P., Vemuganti, G.K., et al.: Early results of penetrating keratoplasty after cultivated limbal epithelium transplantation. Arch Ophthalmol 123, 334–340 (2005)
55. Stoiber, J., Forstner, R., Csaky, D.C., Ruckhofer, J., Grabner, G.: Evaluation of bone reduction in osteo-odontokeratoprosthesis by three-dimensional computed tomography. Cornea 22, 126–130 (2003)
56. Legeais, J.M., Renard, G., Parel, J.M., Serdarevic, O., Mei-Mui, M., Pouliquen, Y.: Expanded fluorocarbon for keratoprosthesis cellular ingrowth and transparency. Exp Eye Res 58, 41–51 (1994)
57. Yaghouti, F., Nouri, M., Abad, J.C., Power, W.J., Doane, M.G., Dohlman, C.H.: Keratoprosthesis: Preoperative prognostic categories. Cornea 20, 19–23 (2001)
58. Lille, S.T., Engrav, L.H., Caps, M.T., Orcutt, J.C., Mann, R.: Full-thickness grafting of acute eyelid burns should not be considered taboo. Plast Reconstr Surg 104, 637–645 (1999)
59. Hagai, T.: Eyelid burns: A general plastic surgeon's approach. In: Hornblass, A. (ed.) Oculoplastic, Orbital and Reconstructive Surgery, pp. 448–454. Williams & Wilkins, Baltimore (1988)
60. Frank, D.H., Wachtel, T., Frank, H.A.: The early treatment and reconstruction of eyelid burns. J Trauma 23, 874–877 (1983)
61. Meyer, D.R., Kersten, R.C., Kulwin, D.R., Paskowski, J.R., Selkin, R.P.: Management of canalicular injury associated with eyelid burns. Arch Ophthalmol 113, 900–903 (1995)
62. Achauer, B.M., Adair, S.R.: Acute and reconstructive management of the burned eyelids. Clin Plast Surg 27, 87–96 (2000)
63. Thai, K.N., Billmire, D.A., Yakuboff, K.P.: Total eyelid reconstruction with free dorsalis pedis flap after deep facial burn. Plast Reconstr Surg 104, 1048–1051 (1999)
64. Gérard, M., Merle, H., Chiambaretta, F., Louis, V., Richer, R., Rigal, D.: Technique chirurgicale de l'autotransplantation limbique dans les brûlures oculaires graves et récentes. J Fr Ophtalmol 22, 502–506 (1999)

Emergency Treatment

Joël Blomet, Lucien Bodson, and Max Gérard

9.1 Characteristics and Consequences of Chemical Ocular Traumas

Chemical trauma is characteristic in that the chemical product is immediately active in contact with tissue, and that its action stops when its concentration drops below its limit of action, which depends on the type of chemical reaction and the energy potential of the chemical aggressor (See Chap. 3).

For the contact time, the chemical agent physically migrates into tissue and can pass through the cornea in 90 s if 4% soda (1 N/pH = 14). Penetration is gradual and induces no immediate deleterious effect. As set out in Chap. 5, cells can survive for some time in contaminated medium. The shorter this time, the greater the chances of cell survival.

Now, for a long time, the lumping together of the mechanisms of thermal and chemical burns has led to erroneous interpretation of observed objective facts.

While rinsing with water will cool deep into the tissue of a thermal burn, rinsing the tissue with water or physiological solution very quickly removes the product but only from the eye surface. Contrary to generally accepted ideas, and as demonstrated by Laux as early as 1965, Josset in 1986 and, more recently, Schrage with his EVEIT® model, rinsing with water or physiological solution does not remove the chemical that has penetrated. Laux had supplemented these data by showing that you had to wash for more than 9 h continuously to achieve a significant effect with water, and still more than one hour and a half with a phosphate buffer.

This penetration dramatically complicates the work of emergency and first aid teams. In fact, as long as the chemical is not really removed from the tissue, the burn can progress (as with alkalis) and will greatly complicate care and healing by disturbing the expected biological cycles.

9.2 Chemical Emergency: A Race Against the Clock

As should by now be obvious, early and effective rinsing is one of the keys to minimizing chemical injuries.

To optimize this rinsing, you have to put the actual action of the chemical contact and the kinetics of tissue penetration in perspective.

As has been seen before, chemical contact depends on the reactivity of the chemical, its reacting force, and especially its physical form.

Liquids are the most quickly reactive. They easily spread over the surface (see the key time in a publication by Schrage), reach into the conjunctival fornices, then penetrate. The eye-closing reflexes accelerate this diffusion. A hydrophobic liquid usually penetrates less quickly than a hydrophilic liquid due to protection by the lacrymal fluid.

Gases are nearly as quick and are slowed down by the time of assimilation into the lacrymal fluid. They dissolve in the tears and behave as an aqueous phase for hydrophilic gases, such as chlorine or ammonia. On the other hand, hydrophobic gases need to mechanically

J. Blomet (✉)
Research Director, Prevor Laboratory, Moulin de Verville, 95760 Valmondois, France
e-mail: jblomet@prevor.com

L. Bodson
Emergency Manager, CHU - ND des Bruyères Université de Liège, Rue de Gaillarmont, B-4030 LIEGE 3, Belgique
e-mail: l.bodson@chu.ulg.ac.be

M. Gérard
Medical director of Head and Neck Unit, Ophtalmologist, Cayenne Hospital, Cayenne, French Guiana
e-mail: gerardmax@caramail.com

work their way through the lacrymal fluid before penetrating the eye. Therefore, their properties are closely dependent on gas miscibility. Vapors and sprays behave much like gases. This explains the delay effect observed with some hydrophobic gases, such as mustard gas.

Solids have a delay effect because they need to dissolve in the lacrymal fluid before reacting with the cornea. A solid form will aggravate the contact not only by its remanence at depth but also by the difficulty of extraction.

Lastly, some relatively trivial bodies from the standpoint of burns, such as a metal chip, cause an oxidization reaction, which attacks tissue and can also lead to a troublesome injury. A solid complicates first aid because its delay effect prevents it from being identified as a chemical agent. The trouble caused by the presence of the solid body is not always sufficient to trigger care appropriate to the chemical.

Thus, the chemical acts in two steps. The first step is surface contact with spreading. This depends not only on form and viscosity for liquids but also on solubilizing power for gases and solids. After this first step, which can be very quick for corrosive products, about 10 s, there is a second step: penetration.

Penetration first depends on the reactivity of the product. Its molecule is accelerated by the energy released during reaction with the antagonists of the cornea, such as the amino acids. This penetration is slowed down by the stericity of the molecules and depends on its lipophilic and hydrophilic character. Consumption during the reaction reduces the penetration depth, as for acids, without however preventing penetration of all the ions. Thus, for hydrofluoric acid, the superficial part will slow down the penetration of the H^+ ion without preventing penetration of the F^- ion. As shown by Schrage, this penetration is accompanied by an increase in osmotic pressure, which will complicate the rinsing. In fact, rinsing with a hypotonic solution like water will create a flow of liquid to rebalance the osmotic pressures from the outside to the inside, favoring the penetration of the ions instead of stopping them.

The early the rinsing, the least need to counter the penetration effect.

While it can be considered that mechanical rinsing, through entrainment and dilution, is really effective to remove a product from the surface, things are quite different for product within tissue, where there is no mechanical effect any more.

The capability to extract the chemicals is essential for effective rinsing. The hypotonicity of water or isotonicity of physiological solution makes these methods contraproductive by preventing the product to come out because of the influence of flows due to osmotic pressure. Hypertonicity cannot alone bring out the products. Active molecules, such as Diphoterine® or Hexafluorine®, are necessary to fully wash off a chemical.

Proper rinsing of the cornea, without omitting the conjunctival fornices, is generally sufficient for liquids. Solids are more paradoxical. Rinsing accelerates their dilution and transforms them into a liquid, provided they are miscible in the rinsing liquid, which is not generally so with metal. If a solid, such as a soda flake, represents the highest concentration at the point of contact, it is actually less dangerous than it appears because only the surface soda that dissolves participates in the burn. Continuous rinsing of the solid during dissolution usually prevents the burn from being severe. A solid is dangerous only by its contact surface, and of course, its contact time.

Two characteristic times can be identified in the analysis of accidents. For the most corrosive products, penetration starts after the first 10 s. This penetration is nearly total after 1 min. The symptoms and their occurrence depend on the seriousness and reversibility of the corrosive or irritating product and its concentration.

9.3 Stakes in the Management of First Aid

There are several stakes in the management of first aid, depending on circumstances. The ideal is to be able to protect the eye by preventing any penetration of a corrosive agent. If action is taken after penetration has begun, the objective becomes to stop penetration and remove the chemical to be able to administer care according to the symptoms observed.

While the conditions of the burn depend only on the chemical, management depends on environmental factors and carers' qualification.

Whatever the situation, the main objective is to remove the chemical as quickly as possible from the eye to lower its aggressive concentration.

Five primary sets of circumstances can be identified.

9.3.1 In Occupational Environments

The risk may have been pre-identified and suitable emergency facilities may have been pre-positioned. This is planned before the accident and makes it possible to take action during the first 10 s and generally avoid the consequences of chemical splashes, even with solids. The use of an active rinsing solution in lieu of water is a key to success. If the risk is multifaceted, it is essential to have polyvalent solutions, such as Diphoterine®, in order not to waste time in identifying the burning agent. A wrong specialist solution could aggravate the problem.

9.3.2 After an Accident on the Public Highway

The lack of suitable emergency facilities and, often, of qualified staff may lead to situations that get complicated. Recommending quick rinsing with water and training the population is one of the keys to facilitating subsequent treatment. The accident at home follows this scheme unfortunately too often. Following misuse by a child or because of mishandling, it is highly regrettable that families are not aware, as in industrial environments, of the hazards posed by household products and of what to do in case of splashes.

9.3.3 Industrial Accidents

Accidents, such as that in Bhopal or the explosion of an ammonia lorry in Dakar, involve a very large number of casualties. The time to set up the emergency services and the complexity of a 15-min rinse with water require the use of active solutions to reduce the time to action and expect a sufficient reliable effect by stopping the action of the chemical, pending possible management in suitable hospital facilities.

9.3.4 Attacks

They can be likened to industrial accidents, by the number of casualties and their unexpected nature associated with everyday life, such as in the underground or in department stores, or during special events, such as sporting events or big concerts. In this case, emergency facilities are always prepositioned. The use of an active positive solution avoids having to identify the product, which delays management too much, and stops the aggressive action of the product before appropriate treatment. The advantage of polyvalent solutions is that they can be used easily and delegated to nonspecialists, if necessary.

9.3.5 Lack of Initial Care

Finally, there is a case where the injured has not been administered care before arrival at the hospital, which may be several hours after the accident. If the symptoms unfortunately appeared and progressed, it is absolutely necessary to stop the action of the chemical before initiating treatment. Polyvalent active solutions, such as Diphoterine®, are the most effective solutions to stop the chemical, avoid aggravation, and consider secondary therapy under the best possible conditions.

9.4 Organizing the Emergency Chain

The keys to successful management of a chemical casualty are the following:

- Early rinsing reduces complications, and action during the first 10 s is ideal. Action during the first minute will usually avoid complications with a polyvalent active solution.
- Water rinsing complicates emergency aid when there are a large number of casualties because of its ineffectiveness and the amounts necessary for a 15-min rinse.
- Whatever the time between the accident and management, effective rinsing is always essential to be able to administer suitable care thereafter. Stopping the action of the chemical and removing it is key to successful subsequent treatment.
- The risk assessment and prepositioning of emergency facilities, as well as personnel training in occupational environments will usually avoid disasters, because management can be very quick.
- Training the population into the need for early rinsing increases the chances of success.
- The need for identifying the chemical is always a waste of time, which delays the critical effect of rinsing.
- Calling specialist structures as early as possible reduces the time of action of the dangerous product.

The organization of the emergency chain should answer the following questions on:

1. The number of persons involved
2. The awareness of the risk
3. The possible prepositioning

The answers then follow the following decisional scheme:

	Awareness of the risk		
	Yes (Occupational environments, D.I.Y.)	No (Accident on the public highway, attack, late arrival at the emergency department)	
		Prepositioned	Non-prepositioned
A few people involved	Organization and staff training with suitable solutions. Polyvalent solutions for safe first care. The response time of less than 10 s is a success factor. The use of amphoteric solutions improves the final prognosis	Effective rinsing can be easily organized with polyvalent solutions. An active hypertonic solution will stop penetration	Advise immediate water rinsing and conduct effective rinsing when medical management is possible
Many people		Only effective rinsing with solutions that stop the action of the chemical is possible	

9.5 Treatment of Ocular Injury: The Importance of the Emergency Chain for Care

9.5.1 Emergency Chain Definition

The emergency chain, in the management of chemical splashes in the eye both in occupational and domestic environment is that allowing quick and coordinated management of any type of emergency to limit morbidity or mortality.

In traumatology, it is easy to understand that any delay in management can but aggravate the injuries, all the more as the aggression is "persistent," as that due to a corrosive chemical. In such a situation, each lost second results in longer contact with the human tissue. The chemical injury aggravates with a real risk of very quick loss of tissue vitality.

Broadly, the emergency chain involves:

1. Early alert
2. Suitable first care
3. Specialist care, if necessary

In a traumatic situation that is not immediately life-threatening, a "response sheet" such as the following can be proposed:

1. Quick recognition of the type of problem and alert
2. Action to remove the risk or move away from the risk
3. Detailed care protocols

9.5.2 Safety Obligations

The safety of witnesses and first aiders is essential. That is why, during missions of the mobile emergency medical services, the first fundamental gesture is that which ensures the safety of the team.

Therefore, in any emergency, whatever its seriousness, the practical and effective sequence will always be of the following type:

1. Quickly recognize the type of problem and, if possible, the precise nature of the risk to trigger a first "simple" alert level.
2. Shield the victims and response persons from the risk or move them away from the risk.
3. Alert the emergency medical care services (112, emergency number in Europe).
4. Administer first care or have first care administered or, if necessary, send the victim to structures that may make more specific diagnostic reviews and decide the implementation of specialist care.

Chemical risk is usually quickly recognized but often more easily and quickly in occupational environments than in domestic environments, less "trained" in this type of situation.

Removing the risk or moving away from the risk is, unfortunately, easier to say than to do. Contrary to "fire or explosion" risks, which are more visible and brutal, chemical risks are more insidious. However, when they are recognized, only quick reaction will affect mortality and morbidity.

For the irritating or corrosive chemicals we are concerned with here, the top priority is to break the "product–human tissue" contact. This can be done in two ways:

- Through spontaneous mechanical entrainment by the victim or by the witnesses: wiping, washing with copious amounts of water
- By fully neutralizing the product by chemical means ("antidote effect")

9.5.3 The Specific Management of Chemical Injuries

Any attempt to administer care after an accident or chemical aggression is doomed to failure if it is impossible to "remove" the aggressive product (or move away from it).

On the other hand, any procedure and any "neutralizer" that prevents or effectively reduces the time of contact with the eye as soon as the chemical nature of the aggression is recognized will be beneficial.

Therefore, it is obvious that, to apply these principles and use this "neutralizer" as soon as possible, the emergency procedure should be well known to everyone and sufficiently simple. In addition, to avoid any loss of time, the "neutralizer" should always be available near the risk.

Once the aggressive product is "neutralized," in the broad sense of the term, than medical care can begin. In all cases of chemical eye injury, medical advice should be sought as soon as possible.

9.6 Which Care Chain for Optimum Management of Chemical Eye Burns?

The management of chemical eye burns is not the sole concern of the ophthalmologist. It takes often several hours between the burn and the visit to the ophthalmologist. During this time, many treatments have been administered, or most often, not administered because they have not been approved by the specialist. Therefore, at the time of the visit to the ophthalmologist, the prognosis is already settled. Here, we have a vicious circle: the most common vision ophthalmologists have of chemical eye burns is "either it is not serious and it will heal, or it is very serious, and there is nothing we can do." Now, it is the ophthalmologist's expertise which will dictate the course of action to be taken. This biased assessment of the problem led to the implementation of treatment strategies, which are interesting but have limitations.

9.6.1 Immediate Care by "Nonspecialists"

First limitation: immediate care is administered to the victim by nonspecialists, or even non-healthcare people. Now, there has been one dogma in France for several decades: a chemical eye burn means washing with water and, above all, not using anything else, especially no "neutralizing" solutions.

This course of action has unquestionable clinical and experimental arguments but only when action is taken during the very first seconds after the corrosive chemical splash. Water rinsing has only a mechanical action, entraining the chemical out of the eye. Therefore, it will simply reduce the number of potential chemical aggressors on ocular tissue.

After one minute, however, all the experimental studies have demonstrated the ineffectiveness and even harmfulness of eye rinsing with water or with the other isotonic solutes (isotonic to blood). In fact, these aqueous solutions dilute the chemical substance and facilitate the release of the active ions of the corrosive or irritating product. In addition, being hypo-osmolar to the cornea, aqueous solutions create flows from tissue surface to the inside, favoring the penetration of the chemical into ocular tissue (see Chaps. 5 "Physiopathology" and 6 "Eye Rinsing Solutions").

9.6.2 Ophthalmological Management is Often Deferred

This is the second limitation of common treatment strategies. For specialist care to victims of chemical eye injuries, ophthalmologists, especially French ophthalmologists, have developed since quite a long time more or less complex surgical strategies to attend to restore sight to severely burnt people: corneal grafting, limbal autograft or allograft, amniotic membrane grafting, and keratoprosthesis.

9.6.3 Practical Consequences for More Effective Management

In addition to these specialist treatments that are relatively late with the reference to the initial chemical splash, there remains ample room for another treatment objective aimed at avoiding or limiting the immediate seriousness of a chemical eye.

To achieve this aim, you need a real eye burn management chain. In reality, many persons will give aid to the burnt person before he/she meets the ophthalmologist. Therefore, the setting up of an eye burn care chain is possible. The difficulty will be to have persons who are most often unqualified administer initial care. This is possible, on the basis of our experience, under three conditions: a good protocol, suitable training, and technical supervision by healthcare professionals.

9.6.3.1 Develop a Protocol Which Must Be Simple in Every Aspect

- Understandable in view of the desired therapeutic action, in order to gain acceptance by the person who is to use it
- Easy to implement, by simple decision-making because of the absence of any contraindication and side effect
- Easy and very quick to implement

9.6.3.2 Training

Training will be essential for the persons who are to implement the protocol. This training shall be given initially and regularly updated. It will combine theoretical aspects and especially practical situations consistent with the type of risk.

9.6.3.3 Necessary Specialized Supervision

This is the third and last condition to achieve a credible, effective system. The action should be supervised by recognized healthcare professionals, so that it is professionally credible and follow-up can be ensured to take account of the results and improve the relevance and quality of the implemented system.

Index

A

Acidic buffering, 62
Acidic function, 19
Acrolein, 24–25
Active wash, 44–46
Alkylation reaction, 21–22
Allograft, 106–109, 117
American Association of Poison Centers, 10
Amniotic membrane, 106
Aqueous humor, 61
Autograft, 98, 100, 105–108, 117

B

Basal cells, 51–52
Basement membrane, 52
Basic function, 19
Benign ocular burns, 99
Boron trifluoride, 37–38
Bowman's membrane, 52
Buccal mucosa transplantation, 104–105

C

Cataract, 101
Cederoth, 83, 90
Cellular survival, 71
Chelating function, 21
Chemical agents and reactions
    biological and biochemical targets, 29–31
    chemical burn knowledge, 46–48
        chemical burns, 17
        parameters affecting chemical burns, 17
    elementary reactivity, 18
    energetic levels of chemical reactivity
        acid–base scale, 25–28
        irritant, 27
        scales of, 27, 29
    mechanisms of chemical burn
        energy dimension, 33–34
        parameters, 34–39
        risk factors, 39–43
        types of chemical reactivity, 31–33
    modulation, reactivity of molecule
        acetic acid and derivatives, 22–23
        acrolein, 24–25
        hydrofluoric acid, 23
        methylamines series, 24
        phenol, 23–24
    molecular structure, irritant/corrosive, 18–19
    reactive functional groups, irritant/corrosive agents
        acidic function, 19
        alkylation reaction, 21–22
        basic function, 19
        chelating function/complexation, 21
        molecular reactivity and chemical bonds, 22
        oxidizing function, 19–20
        reduction function, 20
        solvent function, 20–21
    types of chemical reactivity, 18
Chemical assault, 11–13, 17, 32
Chemical concentration, 39–40
Chemical emergency, 113–114
    emergency care
        active wash, 44–46
        consequences of passive washing, 44
        dilution and mechanical draining, 43–44
Chemical trauma, 113
Clinical signs
    complications, on ocular surface
        corneal nonhealing, 99–100
        ectropium-trichiasis of, 101
        symblepharons, 100–101
    conjunctival alteration, 98
    corneal edema, 96–97
    corneal ulceration
        superficial punctuate keratitis, 96
    endocular complications, 101
    extraocular signs, 99
    intraocular lesions, 98–99
    perilimbal (conjunctival) ischemia
    alkali, 95, 96
    hyperhemia of, 95
    limbus, 94, 95
        upper conjunctival ischemia, 96
    Roper Hall's Prognostic classification, 97
Cold gaze burns, 67
Collagen lamellae, 52, 53
Conjunctiva
    ischemia, 94–96
    pannus, exeresis, 105
    transplantation, 104
Cornea
    anatomy, 49, 93

burns, mechanism of
    with chemically active foreign bodies, 67–68
    with chemically reactive fluids
        acids, 68
        alkali, 68
        detergents/solvents, 70
        hydrofluoric acid, 70
        peroxides, 68–70
        thermal contact, 67
    calcifications, 90
    edema, 96–97
    histology
        Bowman's membrane, 52
        descemet's membrane, 53
        endothelium, 53–54
        epithelium and basement membrane, 49–52
        limbus, 54–55
        stroma, 52–53
    innervation, 55
    leucoma, 101
    nonhealing, 99–100
    osmolarity, 56, 79, 82
    pathophysiology of
        decontamination on eye, 59–61
        eye burns physiological barriers, 59
        impregnation, 65, 66
        irritation and burn, 64–65
        limits of physiological decontamination, 63–64
        local decontamination, 60–63
    scratched, 90
    transparency, 93–94
    transparency, factors of
        collagen structure, 55
        intraocular pressure, 57
        proteoglycans function, 55
        recovery mechanism of, 56–57
        regulation of hydration, 55–56
        scarcity of cells in stroma, 55
    ulceration, 98
        fluorescein with, 96
        superficial punctuate keratitis, 96
    vascularization, 55
Corrosives
    diffusion of, 40–41
    time of contact, with eye, 41–42

D
Decontamination
    active d, 55
    chemical d, 18, 43–46, 87
    emergency d, 18
    initial d, 9
Deep lamellar keratoplasty (DLK), 108
Descemet's membrane, 53
Dilution and mechanical draining, 43–44
Diphoterine®, 36, 45, 71, 77–84, 87, 115

E
Ectropium–trichiasis, 101
Edema, of cornea, 96–97
Emergency care
    active wash, 44–46
    consequences of passive washing, 44
    dilution and mechanical draining, 43–44
Emergency chain, 116
Emergency treatment
    chemical emergency, 113–114
    chemical ocular traumas, characteristics and consequences, 113
    first aid management, 114–115
    management of chemical eye burns
        care by nonspecialists, 117
        ophthalmological management, 117–118
    ocular injury treatment
        emergency chain definition, 116
        safety obligations, 116–117
Endocular inflammation, 101
Endothelial cells, 53–54
Endothelium, 7, 53–56, 59, 70, 71, 78, 79, 82, 93, 108
Energetic levels
    acid–base scale, 25–28
    irritant power of acids/bases, 27
    scales of chemical reactions, 27, 29
Epidemiology, 9–14
Epidemiology, of injuries
    data limitations and scope
        American Association of Poison Centers NDPS, 10
        burn center/hospital studies, 13–14
        individual publications, 9–10
        occupational burn data, 9
        US Bureau of Labor Statistics data, 10
        work-related injury, 11
    etiology
        chemical substances, 14
        complications of face peeling, 13
        deliberate chemical assault, 11–13
Epithelium, of cornea
    basal cells, 51–52
    intermediate cells, 51
    lacrymal secretion, 49–50
    necrosis, 97
    superficial cells, 50–51
Exothermic reaction, 36
Extraocular signs, 99
Eyelid burns, surgical treatment, 109–110

F
Face peeling, 13
First aid management, 114–115

G
Glucose, 30, 31
Glutathione system, 86–88
Guy de Chauliac, 2

H
Hexafluorine®, 38, 70, 87, 90, 114
Hippocrates Heraclidae, 3
History, of chemical burns and relative treatments, 3–4
    eye burns, classification of, 6
    Guy de Chauliac, 2
    Hippocrates Heraclidae, 3

Index

intensive care revolution, thermal burns and, 4–5
Marcel Legrain, 4
medical treatment, 6
origins, 5–6
reconstitutive concepts, 7
rinsing therapy, 6
skin burns, 5
toxicology and ophthalmology, research in, 6
treatment options, 7
Hydrofluoric acid (HF), 21, 28
burn mechanism, 33
decontamination, 87, 89–90
eye burns with, 70
pH, 26, 27
reactivity of, 23
rinsing therapy
decontamination, 87, 89–90
diffusion, 78
Hypertonic, 46, 56, 114

I

Inflammatory mediators
dose response SLS IL-8 from SM, 72, 73
eye burn model, 72
interleukin-8, 72
VEGF
NaOH corneal exposure, 72–73
SLS corneal exposure, 73–74
Innervation, 55
Intraocular lesions, 98–99
Intraocular pressure, 57
Irrigation fluids, rinsing therapy
effect of
anterior chamber pH, 83
buffer capacity, 84
electrolytic contents, comparison of, 83
intracameral pH after corneal rinsing, 85
L929 cell, 85–86
types of, 82
Irritant/corrosive chemicals
molecular structure of, 18–19
reactive functional groups
acidic function, 19
alkylation reaction, 21–22
basic function, 19
chelating function/complexation, 21
molecular reactivity and chemical bonds, 22
oxidizing function, 19–20
reduction function, 20
solvent function, 20–21

K

Keratocytes, 52–53
Keratoplasty
with architectonic goal, 109
lamellar keratoplasty, 108–109
transfixion keratoplasty (TK), 106–108
Keratoprosthesis, 109

L

Lacrymal secretion, 49–50
Lacrymal, 113, 114
L929 cells, irrigation fluids effect, 85, 86
Limbal stem cells (LSC), 105
Limbus
corneal regeneration, 56
epithelial cells, transplantation, 109
histology, 54–55
transplantation
allograft, 106
autograft, 105
conjunctival pannus, exeresis of, 105
Lipids, 30, 31
Liquid metal burns, 67

M

Marcel Legrain, 4
Methylamines series, 24

N

Nasal mucosa transplantation, 104–105
National Poison Data System (NDPS), 10
Necrotic tissues, debridement/excision, 103

O

Ocular anatomy and physiology, 93–94
Ocular hypertonia, 101
Osmolar effect, 78–82
Osmolarity
effects, rinsing therapy, 78–82
eye burns pathophysiology, 70–71
Oxidizing function, 19–20

P

Passive washing, 43–44
Pathophysiology, of eye burns
cellular survival, 71
corneal burns, mechanisms of, 66–70
inflammatory mediators, 72–74
osmolarity, 70–71
penetration characteristics, 71
physiological barriers, 59
Perilimbal ischemia, 94–96
Peroxides, 68–70
Phenol, 23–24
Plum, 83, 84, 90
Pressure, 43
Proteins, 30, 31
buffer, 60
Proteoglycans, 55

R

Reactive functional groups, irritant/corrosive agents
acidic function, 19
alkylation reaction, 21–22
basic function, 19
chelating function/complexation, 21
molecular reactivity and chemical bonds, 22
oxidizing function, 19–20

reduction function, 20
solvent function, 20–21
Reduction function, corrosive agents, 20
Ringler, 81, 83, 84
Rinsing therapy
    development, issues in, 91
    diffusion, mechanisms of, 78
    glutathione system, 86–88
    history, 6
    hydrofluoric acid decontamination, 87, 89–90
    irrigation fluids, effect of
        anterior chamber
        buffer capacity, 84
        electrolytic contents, comparison of, 83
        intracameral pH after corneal rinsing, 85
        L929 cell, exposure of, 85, 86
    osmolar effects in
        blown-up cells, 81
        corneal stroma, 79
        corneal swelling, 82
        cytolysis and necrosis, 120 s of exposure with, 81
        Diphoterine®, 82
        irrigation fluids, types of, 82
        tissue culture, with 800 mOsmol (NaCl), 81
        water contents of, 80
    side effects of
        corneal calcifications, 90
        scratched cornea, 90

S
Safety obligations, 116–117
Sodium lauryl sulfate (SLS), 72–74
Solvent function, 20–21
Stem cell, 71, 91, 95, 96, 98, 100, 104, 105, 109
Stroma, 59, 78-80, 97, 107-109
    collagen lamellae, 53
    corneal regeneration, 57
    ground substance, 53
    keratocytes, 52–53
    scarcity of cells in, 55
    Schwann cells, 53
Sulfuric acid, 39, 40
Superficial cells, 50–51
Supernatant rinsing medium (SM), 72–74
Surgical treatment
    of eyelid burns
        in critical phase, 110

        in sequelar phase, 110
    keratoprosthesis, 109
    lamellar keratoplasty (LK)
        big diameter, 108–109
        deep, 108
    necrotic tissues, debridement/excision of, 103
    symblepharons formation, prevention of, 103
    Tenon's plastics, 103–104
    transfixion keratoplasty (TK)
        big diameter, 106–107
        usual diameter, 107–108
    transplantation
        amniotic membrane, 106
        buccal and nasal mucosa, 104–105
        conjunctival, 104
        cultivated limbal epithelial cells, 109
        limbus, 105–106
Symblepharons, 12, 98, 100, 101, 103, 104, 106

T
Tear fluid, 61
Temperature, 42–43
Tenon's, 55, 103–105
Tenon's plastics, 103–104
Thermal eye burns, 67
Tissue culture, in rinsing therapy
    with Diphoterine®, 82
    with 800 mOsmol (NaCl), 81
Titanium tetrachloride, 36–37
Transplantation
    amniotic membrane, 106
    buccal and nasal mucosa, 104–105
    conjunctival, 104
    cultivated limbal epithelial cells, 109
    limbus, 105–106
Trichloromethylsilane, 37

U
US Bureau of Labor Statistics, 10

V
Vascularization, 55
Vinegar, 22–23
Viscosity, 35–36

W
Work-related injury, 11

Printing and Binding: Stürtz GmbH, Würzburg